C000273793

Phlebotomy

R. F. Hoke

Bsc (Hons) PG Cert HE RODP

Formerly

Clinical Educator
Portsmouth Hospitals NHS Trust

Visiting Lecturer
University of Portsmouth
School of Health and Social Care

First published in Great Britain 2015

Reprinted 2016

By R.F. Hoke
Portsmouth
hoke@btinternet.com

In collaboration with the
National Association of Phlebotomists
London. EC1R 5HL.

A catalogue record for this book is available from the British Library

ISBN 978-0-9933140-0-1

Typeset in Georgia 10 pt
Printed and bound in the United Kingdom

For
David Clements
and
Ben Clements

CONTENTS

ACKNOWLEDGMENTS

I am extremely grateful to Jacqui Hough, Cathy Williams and Jessie Harris from the National Association of Phlebotomists for inspiring me to write this text.

Also, I am indebted to James Stephens from London, who very kindly and expertly, revived my computer, enabling me to retrieve several 'lost' chapters and diagrams. Without his wizardry this text might never have been finished.

I would also like to thank my past students for making phlebotomy interesting and last but by no means least, the many phlebotomists who, with little recognition for their skills, strive on a daily basis to provide and maintain consistently high standards.

Roger Hoke.
May 2015

INTRODUCTION

1

The word phlebotomy is derived from the Greek word *phlebos* meaning 'vein' and the Latin suffix *tome* meaning 'to open'. Originally, the term was used to describe the ancient practice of bloodletting, which remained a popular 'treatment' for many centuries – from the times of the ancient Greeks and Egyptians to the nineteenth century. It is therefore one of the oldest medical practices known.

For around three thousand years, eminent physicians of the day held blood-letting in the highest regard and prescribed it for almost every known ailment including headaches, haemorrhage and fevers. The latter, usually required copious amounts of bleeding – very often on a daily basis until, either the fever subsided or the patient perished.

If the patient survived and was 'snatched back from the jaws of death' this was attributed to the physician's art in knowing just how much blood to draw off, from where, and when. If the patient died, the physicians in their defence would argue that the patient could have survived if only they had been called upon to perform phlebotomy earlier.

In ancient Greece, without knowing that bacteria even existed, let alone caused disease, and unaware that blood circulated, bloodletting was based on two assumptions. Firstly, it was assumed that health and disease were attributable to the balance of four fluids or humours of the body namely, blood, phlegm, black bile and yellow bile. Secondly, they held a strong belief that blood was made from the 'goodness' of food and drink and if not 'used up' blood could stagnate. This gave rise to the term 'bad blood' – an expression still in use today.

Based on the available 'scientific' knowledge at the time, it was hypothesised that a balance of these humours produced health whilst an imbalance caused disease. As blood is the most abundant of these fluids, it was considered the most dominant and therefore the one in most need of re-balancing. To do this, the physician would cut a vein open with a lancet and allow the blood to flow freely into a receptacle. The greater the imbalance, the more blood that would need to be removed – often until the patient collapsed.

Various methods and sites were employed – the most common being the large veins of the arm but also included the backs of the hands, feet and groin or wherever the stagnant blood was believed to lie. Occasionally, it was considered necessary to bleed patients from an artery - although this invariably proved disastrous.

Later, a newer method called *scarification* was introduced which employed a small box containing up to twelve small blades to cut the skin before attaching specially designed glass or china vacuum cups. Because this method required special devices which were not always available, leeches proved a very popular alternative. Other humoral imbalances could be regulated by using purgatives, emetics, or diuretics or in combination – occasionally supplemented with a little blood-letting for good measure.

Phlebotomy was also performed by barbers who had easy access to sharp instruments such as cut-throat razors. The barbers were able to do this without risk of being charged for assault provided they were acting under 'doctor's orders'. Barbershops today still occasionally display the familiar red and white striped pole sign, which originally, was used to signify blood and bandages and advertise their ability in this field.

Blood-letting is only performed in modern practice to treat blood diseases such as haemochromatosis – a condition where the body stores too much iron. By removing some of the iron-rich blood, iron levels are able to return to more normal limits.

Phlebotomy Today

Phlebotomy is often underestimated in terms of its importance to clinical investigations, diagnosis and treatment. Most hospital patients and many attending GP Practices will have blood samples taken as a routine for a variety of indications, all of which are important aspects of patient care. This demands the greatest accuracy and attention to detail and the ability to correctly match the sample to the patient to avoid potentially serious clinical errors.

Modern phlebotomy encompasses a small but important body of specialist knowledge, clinical skills and competencies. It requires a sound knowledge of basic health and safety, infection control, and an appreciation of laboratory requirements. The phlebotomist is also required to possess several important interpersonal skills such as communication, compassion and respect for the patient.

Communication – Practitioners must be able to communicate effectively with patients who may for example have impaired hearing, learning or language difficulties. Good communication skills and the ability to listen are also needed when engaging with colleagues and other healthcare staff such as members of the nursing or medical team.

Body language or non-verbal communication and tone of voice play a significant role in communication and have a greater impact than spoken words alone. It is important that all three convey the same message. Where these are in conflict, non-verbal communication is the most influencing factor.

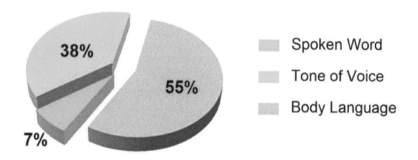

Chart 1. Pie chart showing effect of the spoken word, tone of voice and body language in communication *(7% -38% - 55% rule – Albert Mehrabian).*

Compassion and Respect – Many patients may be suffering from considerable physical pain or discomfort following surgery or illness. The ability to show understanding and respect will always be appreciated by the patient and is the hallmark of professionalism.

Modern Problems in Healthcare

Modern medicine and the changing world have also brought modern problems. By necessity, these have increased the intellectual demands placed on the phlebotomist. Methicillin Resistant Staphylococcus Aureus (MRSA) and Clostridium Difficile (*C. Diff.*) have become very real concerns in hospital wards and departments.

Other diseases such as Human Immuno-deficiency Virus (HIV), Hepatitis B, Hepatitis C, Hepatitis D, new variant Creutzfeldt-Jakob Disease (vCJD), Severe Acute Respiratory Syndrome (SARS) and the outbreak of Ebola virus bring new challenges and the accompanying health and safety risks - not just to the staff member but also patients, their families and visitors.

Training in Phlebotomy

Phlebotomy training in the United Kingdom has always been extremely variable – ranging from the provision of formal study days in some hospitals to simple 'on-the-job' training in others with differences between hospitals and community practices even within the same geographical area.

Although it is the competency which is the most important aspect, a structured training program which enables individuals to understand the process is more satisfying for phlebotomy staff and with greater understanding, may lead to better compliance with policies and guidelines.

Unfortunately, at present there is no nationally regulated training program and syllabus or training validation body – only a national competency standard - *CHS132.2012 Obtain venous blood samples* which is available from the Skills for Health website.

The competency was originally compiled by the NHS – National Patient Safety Agency (NPSA) in their *'Right patient, right blood'* campaign and was entitled *'Obtaining a venous blood sample'* developed in collaboration with Skills for Health.

As part of the campaign the NPSA issued a Special Practice Notice (SPN 14 – November 2006) which required all staff who have a role in the blood transfusion pathway – including those who obtain blood samples, to be competency assessed against this standard every three years. Self-assessment is not acceptable.

This competency has now been updated and is a National Occupational Standard (NOS). Future revisions to the competency and assessment framework will be led by Skills for Health and the Welsh Blood Service Better Blood Transfusion team (Wales).

Some hospitals or NHS Trusts may choose to continue using the NPSA version while others may prefer the updated format or choose to compile their own.

Phlebotomy therefore is inextricably linked by European Directives and national policies and guidelines to the blood transfusion services. Unfortunately when training new staff in phlebotomy, many institutions teach it side-by-side with venous cannulation possibly on the assumption that because both procedures involve needles and veins they require the same skills. Indeed, nothing could be further from the truth.

Cannulation is concerned with inserting a fine plastic tube into a vein for the purpose of administering blood or blood products, fluids or intravenous medication. The cannulae may remain in situ for up to 72 hours before replacement is required. The priority in inserting a cannula is to do so under a strictly aseptic technique to prevent infection and thrombophlebitis caused by the harsh alkaline or acidic interaction between the infusate and the delicate cells lining the walls of the vein.

In phlebotomy the emphasis is on obtaining a sample which is truly representative of the patient's pathology. It must be free from artefacts introduced during the sampling and post sampling stages, correctly labelled and accurately matched to the patient's identification details. The fact that a needle is inserted into a vein for both procedures is purely coincidental.

When phlebotomy and cannulation are taught together it becomes easy for the important aspects of both these skills to be lost so that neither is taught to its full advantage and successful phlebotomy is measured only in terms of whether a sample of blood has been collected in a tube. This can only serve to weaken the patient safety campaigns from organisations such as the NPSA, the Serious Hazards Of Transfusion (SHOT) and other agencies.

Despite the increasing use of technology to identify patients, mistakes still occur and incidences where the sample contains another patient's blood (Wrong Blood In Tube) have increased considerably in the last few years. To turn this trend around a standardised system of quality training and competency assessment is essential.

If we do not rise to the challenge to provide our patients with these most basic requirements for blood specimens then the samples we collect, become meaningless and we will have progressed no further than the ancients and their practice of blood-letting.

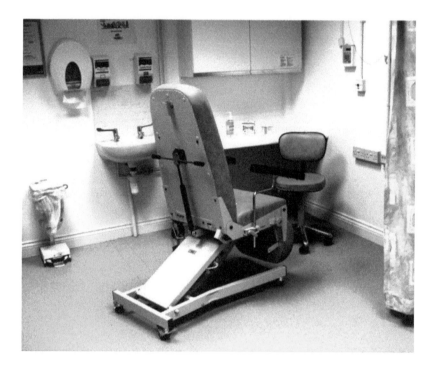

Figure 1. A bright, modern phlebotomy room.

References and Further Reading:

1. CHS132.2912 Obtain venous blood samples. Available from –
   https://skillsforhealth.org.uk   Accessed December 2014.

2. NRLS – NPSA Competency: Obtaining a venous blood sample.
   Available online from –
   http://www.nrls.npsa.nhs.uk/resources/collections/right- patient-
   right-blood/   Accessed December 2014.

3. NPSA. Right Patient, Right Blood. Safer Practice Notice 14.
   http://www.nrls.npsa.nhs.uk/resources/collections/right- patient-
   right-blood/   Accessed December 2014.

2   LEGISLATION

Clinical practice is regulated by a variety of Statutory Acts, policies and guidelines designed to protect patients from harm and abuse. These items of legislation are encountered, often unknowingly, on a daily basis through the numerous interactions staff have with patients, relatives, employers, colleagues, governing bodies and the law. For the vast majority of the time these interactions pass without complaint and are otherwise uneventful.

However, many patients are now aware that they are entitled to have an expectation of standards and level of care and therefore, there is an ever increasing potential for formal complaint and litigation. To ensure that these daily interactions remain uneventful, a basic working knowledge of these legal issues and their application is essential. The problem is that much of the legislation is closely linked so that a study of one aspect reveals a need to have an understanding of another.

Accountability

In simple terms, accountability arises from an agreement or contract where a *principal* (the employer) authorises an *agent* (the employee) to act on their behalf. The principal delegates responsibility to the agent. These agreements occur in several ways.

◆ The patient establishes an agreement by consenting to examination or treatment.

◆ Employers set up an agreement by their employment contract. This is usually supplemented by various policies and guidelines.

◆ Regulatory or governing bodies form an agreement by maintaining a register of qualified and competent members and demanding they comply with their Code of Conduct and Code of Practice.

We are accountable to –

◆　The patient

◆　The Hospital or Employing Health Authority

◆　Professional Organisations

◆　The Law

1. The patient – we are accountable to the patient under civil law where it can be shown that a *Duty of Care* exists. Claims for negligence are usually brought to court by the patient or their relatives and are based on the following criteria:

1.　A relationship must exist that establishes a *Duty of Care*.

2.　This duty of care must have been breached due to the unreasonable acts or omissions of the healthcare worker.

3.　The healthcare worker must have caused the injury, loss or damage.

4.　Action must be brought within a specified period of time known as the Limitation Period. Usually this is three years.

2. The Hospital or Employing Authority – A condition of the employment contract will be that the practitioner always works within their level of competency, follows orders and instructions and safeguards good practice. Where untoward incidents occur to patients, the employer must carry out a full investigation and may be duty bound in some instances to inform professional organisations and suspend or limit the practitioners role until the matter is resolved.

3. Professional Organisations – where the practitioner is a member of a professional organisation, the organisation will have a professional Code of Conduct and a Code of Practice. They will expect members to be honest and trustworthy and competent in their field. Where there is a breach of these Codes, the organisation may seek to suspend the practitioner or for more serious breaches, remove their name from the register preventing any further clinical practice.

4. The Law – this includes several Statutory Acts such as-

- ◆ *Health & Safety at Work Act*
- ◆ *The Mental Capacity Act*
- ◆ *The Mental Health Act*
- ◆ *The Data Protection Act*
- ◆ *The Blood Safety and Quality Act 2005.*
- ◆ *Health and Safety (Sharp Instruments in Healthcare) Regulations 2013*

This section also includes criminal law which protects patients from being deliberately harmed or abused (whether actual or attempted) and covers a wide range of offences for which the perpetrator may be arrested.

Whilst civil law usually seeks financial compensation, criminal law seeks punishment.

Duty of Care

Duty of care requires you to consider the consequences of your actions to ensure that your *acts or omissions* (the things you did but shouldn't have done or the things you should have done but didn't) do not cause a foreseeable risk of injury, loss or damage.

Negligent acts are not intentional nor intended to cause harm but in the eyes of the law they are foreseeable. To fulfill our duty of care we must act as a 'reasonable' person would, taking into account specific skills, knowledge and experience.

If at any time you believe you have made a mistake, it is your duty to inform your supervisor immediately: the sooner you do, the sooner it can be rectified and the safer patients will be. Although no one likes to admit failure, failing to report an error that you are aware of is a deliberate attempt to conceal and is an even bigger mistake.

Remember, mistakes and errors will always occur at some stage. When they do, collectively we learn from them. Existing systems and policies are reviewed or amended to prevent these incidents from happening again.

The Bolam Test

In 1957 the court case of *Bolam v. Friern Hospital Management Committee* became a test of 'reasonableness' in standards of care and skill.

In the case, the patient (the plaintiff) had been given electro-convulsive therapy (ECT) which was widely used at the time to treat depression and schizophrenia. During the convulsion, the plaintiff received a fracture which, during a natural convulsion or fit would be highly unusual and perhaps even more so during a medically induced one. Some doctors used a muscle relaxant as part of the anaesthetic to reduce the severity of the convulsions – others did not. The plaintiff claimed that the doctor had been negligent in that the fracture would not have occurred if a muscle relaxant had been administered.

In summing up the judge, Mr. Justice McNair ruled –

'The test is the standard of the ordinary skilled man exercising and professing to have that special skill. A man need not possess the highest skill at the risk of being found negligent. It is a well-established law that it is sufficient if he exercises the ordinary skill of an ordinary competent man exercising that particular art.'

In other words, a practitioner is not guilty of negligence simply because they are not the best in their field.

However, it is important that practitioners do not extend beyond their level of competence. To do so *is* negligence. Whenever in doubt, seek advice from your manager or a more experienced colleague.

As this case demonstrates, more than one method of practice may be considered correct if each is supported by a body of expert opinion. Practitioners are not negligent simply because there is a body of opinion that takes a view to the contrary. However, where substantiated proof shows a method is outdated, inaccurate or dangerous, the practitioner must update their clinical skills.

Patients or their relatives may bring civil actions not only where they believe the practitioner was negligent but also where they believe the practitioner had been acting without consent and in doing so, had committed common assault or battery.

Vicarious Liability

In the event of an incident where the patient or family members are seeking financial compensation, they will sue the hospital or employing authority as these organisations have overall legal liability and the insurance to pay compensation - either through the NHS Litigation Authority or private insurers. Action against a staff member is rare because even if a court awarded compensation in favour of the plaintiff, it is unlikely that the defendant would have the necessary financial means to pay.

The hospital Trust or employer being the principal, has in law *vicarious* or substituted liability on the employee's behalf. Employers will rightly expect staff to follow good practice guidelines and hospital or departmental policies.

Where these have been breached, they may hold the employee accountable and take disciplinary action against the staff member. This may be in the form of a disciplinary hearing or in extreme circumstances the individual concerned may be suspended from duty or dismissed.

The hospital or employer also has a duty of care. Where a clinical error has occurred or would have occurred, where serious harm or death of a patient was likely, the employer is duty bound to notify the police for the incident to be investigated.

The purpose of this is to determine whether the incident resulted from clinical error where liability may be accepted or whether the incident was due to a deliberate criminal act. This process identifies healthcare staff like Nurse Beverly Allitt and G.P. Harold Shipman and prevents further criminal acts being carried out against patients.

Responsibility

In addition to accountability, we have a responsibility to our employers, our patients and the public to ensure that the provision of care meets acceptable standards and to report to managers when this is not occurring.

When standards fall below acceptable levels healthcare providers can be held to account. This is regulated through a variety of means such as Patient groups and forums, Primary Care Teams, Patient Advisory Liaison Services (PALS) the Care Quality Commission and through Parliament.

Consent

Before undertaking any form of healthcare, the patient's permission must be obtained. Legally, ethically and morally, patients must have the right to decide what happens to them. The process of seeking valid consent is therefore essential in all forms of healthcare. This includes consent for physical examination, diagnostic tests and treatment. Importantly, if the concept of consent is to have any validity or meaning, patients must have the option to refuse.

Consent may be given verbally by direct speech, non-verbally by simply holding out an arm or nodding the head (implied) or in writing and is a continuous process. The patient is entitled to withdraw consent at any time. Continuing after consent has been withdrawn may constitute the offence of battery while to act without consent may constitute common assault.

Providing information to patients in a manner, which they can easily understand, is central to the consent process. Without knowing the benefits and risks, patients are unable to reach an informed choice and therefore give *true* consent. However, the nature of consent goes much further than simply providing information. Therefore, the term **valid consent** is perhaps more appropriate and the one used by the Department of Health.

For consent to be valid, the patient must –

1. Be competent to make the decision.
2. Have received sufficient information in a form they can understand to make an informed choice.
3. Consent of their own free will and not under duress or coerced by healthcare professionals or their family.

Compliance

Where patients give implied consent, staff must ensure that the patient fully understands the principles of the procedure and is giving valid consent and not simply complying with a request. Compliance is the passive submission to the will of another whereas consent is an active process. In other words, a patient may comply with letting you see their arm but they may not consent to having a blood test. It is important to distinguish between implied consent and compliance especially when dealing with patients where there may be difficulties in communication.

Best Interests

Where adult patients lack the mental capacity to give or withhold consent for themselves – whether temporarily or on a permanent basis - no one else can give consent on their behalf although spouses, relatives' and friends should be consulted regarding the patients views. This may reveal their wishes in certain situations for example if they needed a particular operation. Even so, treatment may still be given if it is considered to be in the patient's 'best interests'.

Best interests differ from medical interests as they must take into account the wishes of the patient when competent, their religious and spiritual beliefs and their general health and well-being.

Advanced Directives or Living Wills

A patient may have decided that they would not want a particular operation or treatment in the future, irrespective of the likely outcomes. If this information has been recorded in writing, healthcare staff may be bound by the patient's wishes. The document is sometimes called a *'Living Will'*. (See also Lasting Power of Attorney under the Mental Capacity Act 2005.)

Consenting Teenagers and Children

Teenagers between the age of 16 and 18 years are presumed to have the maturity to give consent for themselves. Importantly, although still minors, they are afforded the same level of confidentiality as an adult and their permission must be sought to disclose information to a parent or guardian.

Some phlebotomy departments now accept younger patients in their early teens without a parent or guardian being present. Although still classed as children they are deemed to be 'Gillick Competent' meaning that in the opinion of a medical practitioner, they have reached a level of maturity which enables them to fully understand the nature of the examination or procedure and give valid consent. Ideally, parental consent will always be obtained wherever possible. Where a competent child gives valid consent to examination or treatment, a parent cannot over-ride the child's decision.

Gillick Competence arises from a Court Case - *Gillick v West Norfolk and Wisbech Area Health Authority and Department of Health and Social Security [1984] Q.B. 581.*

Gillick Competence

The terms 'Gillick competence' and 'Fraser Guidelines' are often used interchangeably as though these terms are synonymous. In fact, they are entirely different. There is also a great deal of miss-information currently being taught as to the facts including the notion that it should now be known as 'Fraser Competence' which is incorrect.

The case was important as the court ruling is now widely applied to many clinical specialities and situations where a child wishes to seek medical advice and treatment without the knowledge or consent of their parents or guardian and where it must be decided whether a child has the maturity to make their own decisions and to understand the implications.

Due to the amount of miss-information currently being circulated, it is worth clarifying the facts by going back to the case which arose in 1980 when the Department of Health and Social Security (DHSS) issued guidance on family planning services for young people. In the guidance it was implied that in certain instances described as *exceptional*, a doctor could lawfully prescribe contraception for a girl under 16 without her parents' consent or knowledge.

In 1982 Mrs Victoria Gillick a mother of five daughters under the age of 16, objected to the guidance and having failed to formally gain an undertaking from the Health Authority that they would not prescribe contraceptives or treatment for her daughters without her consent, she instituted proceedings against West Norfolk and Wisbech Area Health Authority and the DHSS.

The case went to the High Court in 1984 where Mr Justice Woolf rejected Mrs Gillick's claims stating –

"...whether or not a child is capable of giving the necessary consent will depend on the child's maturity and understanding and the nature of the consent required. The child must be capable of making a reasonable assessment of the advantages and disadvantages of the treatment proposed, so the consent, if given, can be properly and fairly described as true consent."

Mrs Gillick took the case to the Court of Appeal where the judges granted in her favour thus reversing the earlier decision. However, in 1985 the DHSS appealed to the House of Lords (Lord Fraser, Lord Scarman, Lord Bridge, Lord Brandon, and Lord Templeman who overturned the appeal and ruled in favour of the original judgement of Mr Justice Woolf.

Fraser Guidelines

Lord Fraser agreed with the appeal by the DHSS on the following provisions –

"...The only practicable course is, in my opinion, to entrust the doctor with a discretion to act in accordance with his view of what is best in the interests of the girl who is his patient. He should, of course, always seek to persuade her to tell her parents that she is seeking contraceptive advice, and the nature of the advice that she receives. At least he should seek to persuade her to agree to the doctor's informing the parents. But there may well be cases, and I think there will be some cases, where the girl refuses either to tell the parents herself or to permit the doctor to do so and in such cases, the doctor will, in my opinion, be justified in proceeding without the parents' consent or even knowledge provided he is satisfied on the following matters:

1. *that the girl (although under 16 years of age) will understand his advice;*
2. *that he cannot persuade her to inform her parents or to allow him to inform the parents that she is seeking contraceptive advice;*
3. *that she is very likely to begin or to continue having sexual intercourse with or without contraceptive treatment;*
4. *that unless she receives contraceptive advice or treatment her physical or mental health or both are likely to suffer;*
5. *that her best interests require him to give her contraceptive advice, treatment or both without the parental consent.*

That result ought not to be regarded as a licence for doctors to disregard the wishes of parents on this matter whenever they find it convenient to do so. Any doctor who behaves in such a way would, in my opinion, be failing to discharge his professional responsibilities, and I would expect him to be disciplined by his own professional body accordingly. The medical profession have in modern times come to be entrusted with very wide discretionary powers going beyond the strict limits of clinical judgment and, in my opinion, there is nothing strange about entrusting them with this further responsibility which they alone are in a position to discharge satisfactorily."

These are known as the Fraser Guidelines. From the text it can be seen that Fraser Guidelines only apply to girls under the age of 16 years seeking contraceptive advice or treatment.

Therefore, when describing a child's ability to understand and consent to general medical investigation and treatment the correct term is 'Gillick Competent'.

In the House of Lords appeal, Lord Scarman's comments in his judgement are often referred to as the test of 'Gillick competency' -

"...it is not enough that she should understand the nature of the advice which is being given: she must also have a sufficient maturity to understand what is involved."

He also commented on parents' versus children's rights:

"parental right yields to the child's right to make his own decisions when he reaches a sufficient understanding and intelligence to be capable of making up his own mind on the matter requiring decision."

England, Scotland, Northern Ireland and Wales are each responsible for their own policies and laws around health and social welfare and have their own child protection system and laws which although they may differ from the English version, they share the same principles.

Confidentiality

Patients have a legal right to confidentiality regarding a variety of matters including their diagnosis, investigations and treatment. No one may divulge any personal details, including to spouses, partners and relatives without the patient's permission. To do so, is a serious breach of patient confidentiality and is always regarded severely by professional bodies and employers. Any breach is always a disciplinary matter. Furthermore, where breaches in confidentiality have occurred the patient may seek legal redress through the courts. The law of confidentiality is built up by precedents from common or case law in previous court judgments' rather than through a specific Act of Parliament.

Phlebotomists can do much to maintain patient confidentiality by ensuring samples and Request Forms are not left where visitors to the ward or department can view identifying details or other information.

Human Rights Act

The Human Rights Act 1998 (HRA98) incorporates into UK law, basic rights which have been set out by the European Convention on Human Rights.

In the Human Rights Act, Article 8 states –

'Everyone has the right to respect for his private life, his home and his correspondence.'

If Article 8 were to be upheld, public bodies like hospitals who breach confidentiality could also find themselves accused of breaching the Human Rights Act.

Data Protection Act

The Data Protection Act 1998 sets out rules for processing personal information and applies to both paper and computer records. The Act requires that data controllers comply with good information handling rules. Much of the information held is private and we have a right to expect it to be secure. Similarly, it is important that because of the information held, we are not confused with someone else – perhaps someone with a similar name or address.

The Data Protection Act requires that personal data is processed fairly and lawfully, is secure, accurate and relevant and is not kept longer than is necessary.

Caldicott - Information Governance

The Chief Medical Officer commissioned a review led by Dame Fiona Caldicott to review the transfer of all patient-identifiable information from one NHS organisation to another or to non-NHS organisations where information is transferred for purposes other than direct medical care, research or where there is a statutory requirement.

The aim was to ensure that current practice complied with the Department of Health's guidance on *The Protection and Use of Patient Information* (March 1996). This was largely in response to the development of information technology at the time and its ability to disseminate information rapidly and extensively.

The principles are –

- Justify the purpose
- Do not use patient-identifiable information unless it is absolutely necessary.
- Use the minimum necessary patient-identifiable information.
- Access to patient-identifiable information should be on a strictly need-to-know basis.
- Everyone with access to patient-identifiable information should be aware of his or her responsibilities.
- Understand and comply with the law.

Caldicott Guardians

A number of recommendations were made in the Caldicott Report (December 1997). In particular –

'A senior person should be nominated in each NHS organisation, including the Department of Health and associated agencies, to act as guardian. The "guardian" should normally be a senior health professional or be closely supported by such a person.'

The Mental Capacity Act 2005

This Act received Royal Assent on the 7th April 2005 and came into full effect in October 2007. Its purpose was to establish in law best practice and common law principles for those who lack mental capacity and those who make decisions on their behalf. Generally, the Act will only apply to those aged 16 or over. It provides a statutory framework to empower and protect all individuals who lack the capacity to make some decisions for themselves and replaces Part 7 of the Mental Health Act 1983 and the whole of the Enduring Power of Attorney Act 1985.

There are five key principles which are set out in Section 1 of the Act.

- **A presumption of Capacity** – all adults have the right to make their own decisions and must be assumed to have the capacity to do so until proven otherwise. It is important to remember that a person may have the capacity to make some decisions but not others.

- **Encouragement to make decisions** – A person is not to be treated as unable to make a decision unless all practicable steps to help him to do so have been taken without success.

- **Individuals must be given the opportunity and support to make their own decisions**. Assumptions of mental capacity should never be made on the grounds of age or disabilities.

- **Individuals must be allowed to make unwise decisions even if the reason may seem irrational.** They must not be considered to lack mental capacity simply because their view differs.

- **Where an act or decision is made for an individual** it should be the least restrictive of their basic rights and freedoms.

The Act also includes three further provisions to protect vulnerable people. These are –

- An Independent Mental Capacity Advocate (IMCA) who will speak for individuals where they do not have family or friends who are able to do so.

- The ability to make advanced decisions to refuse treatment – even if this is life threatening.

- The introduction of a new criminal offence of neglect or ill treatment of someone who lacks mental capacity and is punishable by a term of up to five years imprisonment.

Mental Health Act

Adults are always assumed to be competent unless it can be demonstrated to the contrary. Competent adult patients are entitled to refuse treatment – even where it would clearly be of benefit except when detained under the *Mental Health Act* 1983.

The Act enforces the patient to undergo psychiatric treatment. However, while the patient is unable to refuse psychiatric treatment, they may refuse examination or treatment of an accompanying physical illness. Therefore an adult may be deemed incompetent to make some decisions but competent to make others.

Refusals, for what may appear as totally illogical reasons, do not prove that the patient is incompetent but may be indicative of some underlying fear or anxiety which requires further investigation and discussion.

Employers Policies

Employers have an enormous range of obligations to patients and their employees as well as Statutory Acts and European Directives. To meet these legal requirements, policies and guidelines are necessary to establish a framework for staff to function.

◆ Practitioners must read and follow their employer's clinical guidelines and policies.

◆ Be aware of and follow guidelines from professional bodies

◆ Ensure their practice is current.

◆ Seek advice from a supervisor when in doubt.

◆ Continue professional development.

Health and Safety

The Health and Safety at Work Act 1974 places a duty of care on every employee to take all reasonable steps for the health and safety of themselves and others.

Employees have a duty to follow advice or policies set out by the employer so that the employer is able to meet statutory requirements including those set by the Health & Safety Executive (HSE) RIDDOR (Reporting of Injuries, Diseases and Dangerous Occurrences Regulations 2013) and Control of Substances Hazardous to Health (COSHH).

The Health and Safety (Sharp Instruments in Healthcare) Regulations 2013 came into force on the 11 May, 2013. Under the - *Use safer sharps (incorporating protection mechanisms) – regulation 5(1)(b)* - The employer is required to substitute the traditional, unprotected medical sharps with a 'safer sharp' where this is possible and is reasonably practicable to do so.

The term 'safer sharp' means medical sharps which incorporate features or mechanisms that are designed to prevent or minimise the risk of sharps injury. For example, a range of phlebotomy needles and winged collection sets are available that incorporate a guard or cover which slides or pivots to cover the needle after use.

These safety devices should include a tactile and audible 'click' when the safety guard is activated. This protective guard should not be easily reversible.

Using 'safer sharps' does not of course mean that injury cannot occur: care and vigilance are still very important aspects to safe practice.

References & Further Reading

1. Health & Safety Executive. Health and Safety (Sharp Instruments in Healthcare) Regulations 2013 Guidance for employers and employees. Available from – http://www.hse.gov.uk/pubns/hsis7.pdf Accessed December 2014.

2. Health & Safety at Work Act 1974. Available from - http://www.hse.gov.uk/legislation/hswa.htm Accessed December 2014.

3. Confidentiality – NHS Code of Practice. Available from - https://www.gov.uk/government/uploads/system/uploads/ attachment_data/file/200146/Confidentiality_- NHS_Code_of_Practice.pdf   Accessed December 2014.

4. Mental Capacity Act. Available from - http://www.legislation.gov.uk/ukpga/2005/9/contents Accessed December 2014.

5. National Guidance for child protection in Scotland. Available from -http://www.gov.scot/Publications/2014/05/3052/0

6. Welsh Assembly Government (2007) Safeguarding children: working together under the Children Act 2004 (PDF) Cardiff: Welsh Assembly Government.

7. HM Government (2013) Working together to safeguard children: A guide to inter-agency working to safeguard and promote the welfare of children (PDF).

8. Gillick v West Norfolk and Wisbech Area Health Authority and Department of Health and Social Security [1984] Q.B. 581.

9. Wheeler R. Gillick or Fraser? A plea for consistency over competence in children - Gillick and Fraser are not interchangeable. *BMJ* 2006;332:p807.

10. Payne-James J, Dean P, Wall I. Medicolegal essentials in healthcare. Churchill Livingstone. 1996.

11. Consent to treatment. http://www.nhs.uk/conditions/consent-to treatment/pages/introduction.aspx   Accessed 07/05/2015.

3   BASIC PRINCIPLES

Clinical investigations and health screening tests rely heavily on blood samples to aid the process. The method is generally easy to do, reasonably quick and relatively painless for the patient and minimally invasive. Blood samples are taken for a wide variety of conditions and reasons such as-

- To confirm or eliminate a diagnosis
- Health screening
- Monitor effects of treatment
- Monitor disease progression
- Pre-operative assessment
- Tissue typing (in organ transplantation)
- Blood Transfusion

The risks associated with phlebotomy to patients are through direct and indirect errors.

Directly

- Haematoma
- Arterial puncture
- Trauma to tissues
- Nerve damage
- Infection
- Thrombophlebitis

Indirectly

- Diagnostic and treatment errors
- Transfusion errors including death

All laboratory investigations can be divided into three distinct phases:–

The pre-analytical phase – starts from the time a blood sample Request Form is generated, the sample is obtained by the phlebotomist, and transported to the laboratory. Within the laboratory, the sample details are entered onto the computer system and the sample tube has a bar-code label attached. This phase ends when the analysis begins.

The analytical phase – occurs within the laboratory when analysis commences and ends when the process is complete.

The post analytical phase – begins with the validated results being posted on the computer system, results printed, and the phase ending when the medical or nursing staff review the results.

Each phase is in itself a multi-stage procedure involving numerous members of staff. At each stage and with each worker, there is the potential for an error to occur. Sometimes, more than one error can occur with as many as seven in one incident having been reported in the past.

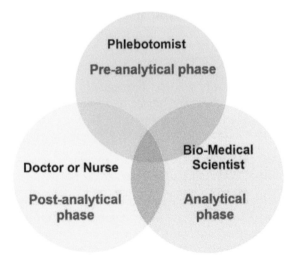

Figure 2. The three phases of an investigation and the staff groups involved. Each is equally important in maintaining integrity of the sample.

An interesting point is that Biomedical Scientists, Doctors and Nurses, having completed university courses, are all registered healthcare professionals. Yet the phlebotomist or healthcare worker, who takes the sample which everyone else will act upon, may only have had the very briefest of training.

From the Venn diagram (Figure 2.) it can be seen that each participant in the collecting, analysing, processing, diagnosing and treating has an equal value. No one member role or task is more important than the others. Collectively, they form a triad - a phlebotomy trinity.

If the phlebotomist obtains the sample from the correct patient, the laboratory will analyse the correct sample and the doctors can make the correct diagnosis and the nurses can deliver the correct treatment.

However, if the phlebotomist were to get it wrong, the laboratory will analyse someone else's blood, accurately report these erroneous results leading the doctors to make a false diagnosis, and the nurses to administer the wrong or inappropriate treatment or medication.

Case Study 1.

The following incident occurred in a six-bedded ward in an NHS Hospital.

Patient A *was due a blood transfusion and a Cross-Match sample was to be taken. A series of errors occurred where the sample was obtained from* **Patient B** *and labelled with the details from* **Patient C**.

There was no record of the staff group (doctor / nurse / Phlebotomist /other staff grade) who took the sample.

Fortunately, the error was identified in the laboratory from an earlier sample and no harm was caused. Had an incompatible transfusion taken place, the consequences for the patient could have been fatal.

This is an example of a Critical Incident which shows how important phlebotomists roles are. This could have been disastrous but for the intervention of someone in the laboratory.

Phlebotomy falls completely into the pre-analytical phase. This may be further divided into three sub-groups –

The Pre-Sampling Stage – This begins when the phlebotomist positively identifies the patient using four points of ID and matching against the ID-band (where applicable) and the Request Form.

The Sampling Stage – begins when the phlebotomist selects and preps the site, applies the tourniquet, performs venepuncture and obtains the sample through to removal of the needle, disposal of sharps and application of the dressing.

The Post-Sampling Stage – includes the labelling, packaging and transportation to the laboratory which should always be in a timely manner. Some specimens will need to be transported in an upright position, kept warm or placed on ice. Never store specimens overnight in a refrigerator as this can cause potassium to leach out of the red blood cells causing an artificially raised level.

Identity Bands (Wristbands)

Between February 2006 and January 2007 the National Reporting and Learning Service received 24,382 reports of patients mismatched to their care or treatment. It has been estimated that more than 2,900 of these reports relate to errors with Identity Bands. This led to a Safer Practice Notice to be circulated to all NHS Trusts to standardise Identity Bands which should be –

◆ White with black text – This should be in a standard font such as Helvetica, Arial or Frutiger Roman and in 12 – 14 point sizes. This allows for easy readability especially for those with visual impairment or for clarity in low light levels such as hospital wards at night.

◆ Patients who have an allergy or who do not wish to receive a blood transfusion or blood products should have a RED identity band but the lettering must still be black on a white background. A red ID band should prompt the healthcare worker to view the patient's notes or speak to the nurse in charge to gain further information.

◆ Patients must only wear ONE Identity Band.

Identity Bands should only include the following core information - Last name, First name, Date of Birth, and NHS number. A temporary number such as a Hospital or Accident and Emergency Department Number can be used where the NHS number is unknown. Too much information such as NHS number, hospital number, District number can all add to the potential of error because it is difficult to know whether all data is correct.

In Wales only, the first line of the address is also required following a Welsh Health Circular.

ID Band Format

LAST NAME	in UPPER case
First name	in lower case
Date of Birth	in DD – Mmm- YYYY where Mmm is the abbreviated month in letters. Single days are preceded by a zero e.g. 03 – Mar - 2001
NHS Number.	In the 3 3 4 number format

Example:

```
NAME:      JAMES,  Thomas
D.O.B:     O3 - Nov - 1953
NHS No:    123 456 7890
```

All patient Identity Bands should:

- Meet the NRLS's design requirements.
- Only include the core patient identifiers.
- Use set colours for wristbands and text.
- Be generated and printed from the hospital demographic system at the patient's bedside, wherever possible.

Pre-printing several labels with patient details, so they can be used as required for the patient's care, is unsafe.

The format used on ID bands should be used whenever handwriting notes as well. By writing the last name in upper case, enables immediate differentiation between those patients who have first and last names which are interchangeable such as Thomas JAMES and James THOMAS.

The date of birth follows the UK format of **day, month, year**. This is important as we live and work in a world where our computers and many overseas staff use the American format of month, day, year. Temporary hand-written wristbands have the potential for the writer to have a momentary memory slip and enter the date in their usual format which could easily lead to miss identification of a patient with a similar name.

Near Miss and Wrong Blood in Tube

Positively identifying the patient by 4 points of ID is one of the most crucial steps in phlebotomy and yet is often, one of the main areas where mistakes occur.

This has led to a number of *'Near Miss'* incidents where the potential existed for patients to receive an incompatible blood transfusion had it not been detected before transfusion occurred.

In the 2013 – 2014 Serious Hazards Of Transfusion (SHOT) Annual Report it was stated that of the 996 near miss reports, 643 (64.6%) were due to *'Wrong Blood In Tube'* (WBIT). Alarmingly, this has increased by 60% over the last 4 years.

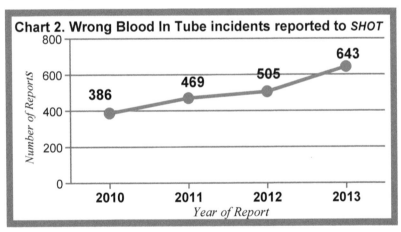

Chart 2. Wrong Blood In Tube incidents reported to *SHOT*

The data shown relates only to blood transfusion samples reported to SHOT. However, as staff taking samples do not deliberately or wilfully mix up transfusion samples, it follows that there must be many more incidences of Wrong Blood In Tube occurring to biochemistry, haematology, virology, immunology and bacteriology samples. It suggests that nationally, the incidence of WBIT is considerably higher than reported and therefore a very real concern.

Over the last decade or so, a great deal of work has been done to reduce this type of error through training and national campaigns such as the National Patient Safety Agency (NPSA) 'Right Patient – Right Blood' together with reports and recommendations from The Serious Hazards Of Transfusion (SHOT).

The introduction of two-dimensional bar-code technology and Radio Frequency Identification (RFID) on hospital In-patient Identity Bands with the ability to print tube labels at the bedside has reduced human transcription errors but has produced one or two other interesting problems.

Case Study 2.

A hospital purchased 2-D Identity Band scanners and printers to prevent mislabelling of sample tubes. Instead of buying a combined, hand held device, separate items were bought. The printers were large and bulky and so were attached to the phlebotomists trolleys.

A phlebotomist attended a patient in a side room but due to the confined space had to leave her trolley (and printer) outside the door. She checked the patient's identity verbally and made a visual check of the ID Band. She then scanned the bar code on the ID Band and the patients details were sent to the printer and held in the printer memory awaiting the phlebotomist's instruction to print the required number of labels.

Unfortunately, the phlebotomist was unable to obtain a sample and marked the form for the doctors' attention. She went on to her next patient in an adjacent side-room and successfully obtained a sample for blood transfusion. Unfortunately, the previous patients details were still in the printer memory and these were printed and attached to the sample tubes. The phlebotomist was unaware that this could happen and as the check was being made by a computer, she felt there was no need for her to double check.

Because the printer had a buffer memory and labels were to be printed after the samples were obtained, the remainder of the phlebotomy round could have been completed with samples labelled in arrears. This type of error is extremely worrying because it could occur to many phlebotomy staff in a hospital and on a daily basis. Until something goes drastically wrong, who would think to query the accuracy of the patients details on the tube? After all, that was the purpose of installing 2-D bar code technology.

Wrong Blood In Tube incidents happen in two main forms-

◆ Blood is taken from the wrong patient and labelled with the correct patient's details

or

◆ Blood is taken from the correct patient but labelled with another patient's details.

To counter this possibility in blood transfusion, many hospitals have implemented a *Two Sample Rule* for blood cross-match. This means that a sample has been previously grouped. A second sample must be sent when cross-matched blood is required. The second sample must be exactly the same blood group as the first sample for a unit of blood to be released.

It is vital that these samples are taken on separate occasions and ideally, by different members of staff. They must never be taken at the same time with one sample held back until the unit of blood is required. Electronic generation of sample labels which include date and time should alert laboratory staff should this occur.

Why Do Things Go Wrong?

Much of the theory around why mistakes happen is attributed to the work of James Reason, Professor Emeritus, at the University of Manchester and his Human Error Theory. This theory has been widely used in industry for many years and forms the basis of the NPSA Root Cause Analysis Tool Kit.

Types of Error

1. Attention Slips and Memory Lapses
2. Mistakes
3. Violations

Attention Slips and Lapses

We all experience these from time to time – we become preoccupied or distracted and something important simply slips our minds.

An example is a nurse colleague who admitted she once sent a sample to the laboratory with her own name and date of birth on the tube! Moments earlier she had been filling out some personal forms which obviously played on her mind and she functioned in repetitive task mode.

Often, many routine and repetitive tasks are performed as 'reflex' actions or reactions and are carried out at a lower level of consciousness. The drawback with operating under these conditions is that our conscious mind wanders onto a subject more stimulating which interrupts the automatic process.

To prevent this pattern of activity, important areas in the sampling procedure should be identified as '*critical points*' such as when checking a patient's identity or labelling samples, giving the phlebotomist the opportunity to refocus on the task. We should not allow colleagues to distract us when 'critical points' are reached, nor distract colleagues when they are carrying out similar 'critical' tasks.

Mistakes

These may be considered by two principle types:

1. **Rule Based Mistakes** – These may occur where rules such as phlebotomy policies or guidelines are too loosely worded so that either the phlebotomist miss-applies the rules or the rules are incorrect. The latter may occur where policies and guidelines are written by staff whose skill or experience is limited or outdated.

2. **Knowledge Based Mistakes** – These can occur where the phlebotomist encounters an unusual situation where their knowledge of policies or guidelines fail to provide them with a rule- based solution. Consequently, any on-the-spot decision is based on a lack of specific information. An example may be where a phlebotomist is asked to take blood cultures. As she has never been shown the procedure she presumes they are taken in exactly the same way as other samples.

Violations

These are the most serious as violations are always deliberate breaches of policy. They may be performed after reasoning or performed routinely as shortcuts by individuals in the belief that their method is much quicker, will save time or money or that it is somehow better for the patients. Sometimes violations can form a common departmental routine to the point that everyone knows what should be done but no one does because they believe the action unnecessary. Many violations are reckless but often carried out in the belief that it bestows some benefit to the patients, their department or hospital. Harm is never intended.

However, these violations are negligent acts or omissions and leave the practitioner and their NHS Trust or other employer who is vicariously liable, open to a charge of negligence.

"Thousands of NHS Samples Mislabelled"

A Freedom of Information Act (FOI) request was sent to every NHS Trust in the UK by More4 News (Channel 4). Of these only 120 replied showing that 365,608 specimens were mislabelled before they arrived at the pathology laboratories.

A further 11,712 samples were also mislabelled in the laboratory by pathology staff.

When labelling samples, especially by hand, remember, all sample tubes must contain 4 points of ID – First Name, Surname, Date-Of-Birth and NHS or Hospital Number plus date, time and signature.

The only exceptions are when taking blood from –

- an unconscious patient in the Accident and Emergency Department

- an un-named new born baby

- Samples taken in the genito-urinary medicine (GUM) clinics where patient anonymity is assured.

Each department will have their own policy and guidelines which must be followed when labelling these specimens.

41

References and Further Reading

1. NRLS – NPSA. Identity bands. Available from -
    http://www.nrls.npsa.nhs.uk/resources/?entryid45=59824
    Accessed: November 2014.

2. Serious Hazards of Transfusion 2014 Annual Report–
    Available from -
    http://www.shotuk.org/shot-reports/
    Accessed December 2014.

3. Reason J. Human Error. Cambridge University Press: 1990.

4. NRLS – NPSA Root Cause Analysis. Available from -
    http://www.nrls.npsa.nhs.uk/rca/   Accessed March 2015.

CHECKING PATIENT IDENTITY 4

One of the most important aspects of phlebotomy is accurately and positively identifying the patient. Our patients place their trust in us and rightly expect their sample to be correctly labelled and matched to their identification details. Indeed, this is a prerequisite for submitting any form of specimen.

Whenever checking a patient's identity, always use 'open' questions. An open question requires the patient to tell you their name. A closed question merely requires a yes or no answer.

The method of carrying out Positive Patient Identification varies depending on whether the patient has been admitted to hospital or is being seen as an out-patient. All hospital in-patients or hospital day-patients' who are to be given treatment such as chemotherapy or blood transfusion, must be wearing a patient identity band or similar method of identification such as a photo-name badge.

This is vital because, if the patient were to collapse or suffer some ill-effect which rendered them unable to speak for themselves, it is the ID Band which speaks for them and is the only positive means of identifying them by their full name, date of birth and NHS or Hospital Number.

Healthcare staff should check and confirm the details of the ID band each time an intervention occurs. This ensures the ID Band contains the correct details and is securely attached to the patient. Where the ID band is missing, blood samples must be withheld until the situation is resolved.

Many staff carrying out identity checks can miss errors because they are looking for confirmation of the identity as opposed to ensuring the information is correct. Remember, someone had to enter the data initially through a computer keyboard and typographical errors can and do occur.

Case Study 3.

*During an ID Band Audit at St. Anywhere's Hospital it was noted that a patient in the Intensive Therapy Unit had an incorrect Hospital Number on their ID Band which did not match the Hospital Number on the patient's notes. The error was simply that a **7** had been substituted for a **1**.*

The ID Band had been in place for at least 11 days and presumably checked numerous times with each nursing and medical intervention.

Interestingly, the hospital Information Governance Department acknowledged that it was busy sorting through 80,000 duplicate entries on its database system.

When checking numbers it is a good idea to verify only three or four numbers at a time.

Because we are only human, we can experience the phenomena where the correct numbers or letters exist but two or more are transposed; when reading through, our brains rearrange them so that we read them correctly. We have probably all experienced this in some form or another – perhaps when typing an email or letter where we fail to notice typographical or spelling errors even though we have read it through, and checked.

This occurs because when reading quickly, we look at the shape of the words not the individual letters.

When checking details, staff should actively look for errors – not simply seek identity confirmation. Read slowly!

When using electronic bar code technology, it is still important to ask the patient to state their name and date of birth and check this against the ID Band. This confirms the patient details on the band are correct. The scan and subsequent printing of labels alleviates transcription errors but a final visual check of the ID Band and labels should still be made. Always read and follow your Trusts Policy and Guidelines.

Figure 3. Checking details on the ID Band accurately match those on the Request form.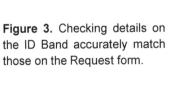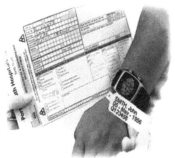

Checking an In-Patients Identity

◆ Approach the patient with a positive and courteous manner.

◆ Introduce yourself stating your role and purpose of visit.

◆ Gain valid consent.

◆ Ask the patient to tell you their full name and date of birth using 'open' questions.

◆ Check the patient's reply against the details on the ID Band.

◆ Clarify any unusual name spelling.

◆ Cross-check the details on the ID Band against the details on the Request form to ensure it is the right patient and not another patient with a similar name.

◆ Scan ID Band (if barcode technology is available).

◆ After obtaining samples, always check label(s) bear the correct patient details before attaching to the sample tube.

◆ Always label tubes at the patient's side taking details from the ID Band if labelling tube by hand.

Checking an Out-Patient's Identity

◆ Approach the patient with a positive and courteous manner.

◆ Introduce yourself stating your role and objective.

◆ Gain valid consent.

◆ Ask the patient to tell you their full name and date of birth using 'open' questions.

◆ Check the patient's reply against the details on the Request Form.

◆ Clarify any unusual name spelling.

◆ Scan Request Form (if barcode technology is available).

◆ After obtaining samples, always check label(s) bear the correct patient details before attaching to the sample tube.

◆ Always label tubes in the presence of the patient – once they have left the clinic it is too late to query any information. If tube labelling is completed by hand, take details from Request Form using a ball-point pen. Gel pens can smudge leaving the details illegible.

Always follow your institutions policy regarding identification of unconscious patients or those who are unable to speak for themselves. They should have an ID Band which must be checked but it is also a good idea for phlebotomy staff when confronted by an unconscious patient to report to the Nurse-in-Charge for further clarification.

Many texts state that sample tubes must be labelled at the bedside but fail to explain why. The reason is simply that in the case of a blood transfusion, where the sample is labelled from the ID Band the information on the sample tube is used by the laboratory to cross-match the unit of blood and these details are on the blood unit label.

When the nursing staff prepare to administer the unit of blood at the patient's bedside, they check the details on the blood bag against the ID Band. If they are a perfect match, the blood is administered.

This way, the same verified information source is used throughout the process – from vein to vein.

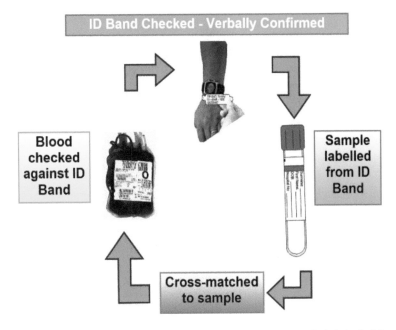

Figure 4. The Blood Sample / Transfusion Cycle. The sample is labelled from the ID Band, cross matched and unit of blood is checked against the same ID Band. All stages use the same source of information and data.

If a sample labelled from the ID Band fails to match the Request Form, the laboratory will reject the sample. However, if the sample is labelled from an incorrect request form, providing the details match, the laboratory may continue to process the sample. One simple failure by the nurse carrying out the bedside check could lead to a patient receiving an incompatible blood transfusion.

The same principle applies to all samples and is the rationale behind the use of two dimensional bar code readers and label printers.

> **Never Use Pre-Labelled Tubes. Only label after the sample has been taken and you have thoroughly checked the details and confirmed patient identity.**

If patients are known to have been issued with an incorrect Identity Band, the Laboratory should be notified immediately as many existing samples may be attributed to the wrong patient.

Case Study 4

At a new junior Doctor's induction, all FY1 doctors were required to demonstrate competency in obtaining a blood sample for transfusion in order to comply with the NPSA Safer Practice Noticed No. 14.

A classroom was set up with a training manikin wearing an ID Band and a hand written Transfusion Request Form appropriately completed with a fictitious patient's details.

The doctors were able to ask the patient to state their name and date of birth and a member of the teaching staff would answer on the imaginary patient's behalf. They then had to check the Hospital Number on the ID Band against the Request Form. If all was correct they were to obtain a sample and label the tube by hand taking the details from the ID Band.

There were three deliberate errors on the form - two involving transposition of numbers (date of birth & Hospital No) and one involving transposition of two letters in the first name.

Of 15 FY1 doctors in the group, only 5 (33%) noticed and queried the errors. All others completed the sample label from the incorrectly hand-written Request Form.

This was set as an experiment to demonstrate to the doctors that when they are busy, tired or distracted, it is easy to see what they expect to see.

The learning outcome was -

Always look for errors not just confirmation because once confirmation is obtained, we stop checking.

BLOOD PHYSIOLOGY

5

Normal circulating blood is composed of three main types of cells: red cells (erythrocytes), white cells (leucocytes), and platelets (thrombocytes).

These cells are suspended in a pale yellow fluid called plasma which contains approximately 90% water and other constituents such as sodium (Na), potassium (K) magnesium (Mg), calcium (Ca), bicarbonate, phosphate, iron (Fe), copper (Cu), iodine (I), and cobalt (Co). Additionally, plasma contains nutrients such as proteins and vitamins, hormones, blood clotting factors, immuno-globulins, antibodies, and gases such as oxygen and carbon dioxide.

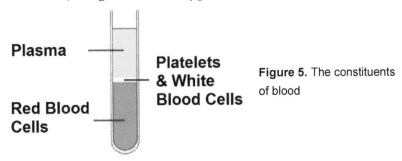

Plasma

Platelets & White Blood Cells

Red Blood Cells

Figure 5. The constituents of blood

Red Blood Cells – these are the most prolific in numbers. Their red colour is due to the pigment *haem* which makes up haemoglobin (Hb) and combined as oxy-haemoglobin, transports oxygen (O_2) from the lungs to the body tissues and returns carbon dioxide (CO_2) to the lungs for elimination. In adults, red cells survive for about 120 days before being broken down in the spleen.

The cells are described as bi-concave discs with a diameter of about 7.2 micrometres (microns). This shape allows the red cells to deform to pass through the smallest capillaries and serves to increase the surface area of the cell, facilitating greater oxygen carrying capacity.

Red Blood Cell

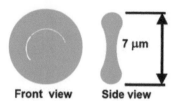

Figure 6. Diagrammatic representation of a red blood cell.

Front view   Side view

White Blood Cells – This is a group of 5 different cell types rather than a specific cell. They are also called leukocytes (*leukos* meaning white). All cells types within the group have a role in fighting bacterial infections.

Neutrophils – these are the most numerous making up 60 – 70% of circulating white cells. They are able to destroy bacteria by ingestion - a process called *phagocytosis* (from the Greek *phago* meaning 'to devour'.

Neutrophils circulate in the blood for about 10 hours before moving into the tissues where they defend tissue cells against bacterial and fungal infections.

Patients receiving chemotherapy often become very depleted of neutrophils (*neutropaenic*) leaving them open to opportunistic bacterial infections. Whenever entering side rooms of neutropaenic patients, remember they are in *Protective Isolation* and thorough hand-washing and the wearing of gloves and aprons is essential. Always check with the nursing staff before entering isolation rooms and follow your hospital's policy.

Lymphocytes – these are the second most numerous white cells making up about 30%. They are produced in large numbers in the lymphatic glands. There are different types of lymphocytes such as T-lymphocytes and B-lymphocytes.

Lymphocytes carry and can produce antibodies as part of the body's immune response to infection.

Monocytes – these cells circulate in the blood stream for approximately 10 hours before moving into the tissues where they develop into macrophages which, like neutrophils, can also ingest bacteria.

Eosinophils – these cells contribute about 1% of circulating white cells. They are named eosinophils because they readily take up the red laboratory stain *eosin*. They circulate for about 5 hours before moving into the tissues. Their main function is to defend against parasitic infections by releasing histamine and helping in allergic response.

Basophils – These have the least numbers of circulating cells making up approximately 0.5%. They have a role in immune responses and are active in anaphylactic reactions.

Platelets – these small, disc-like cells are the second most numerous in the blood and survive in the circulation for about 10 – 12 days. Their main role in conjunction with a number of clotting factors is to arrest bleeding.

Functions of the Blood

- Transport oxygen from the lungs to all tissues and organs
- Transport carbon dioxide to the lungs for elimination.
- Transport nutrients from the digestive system
- Transport hormones secreted by the endocrine glands
- Removal of cell waste
- Circulate antibodies for protection against infection
- Circulate clotting factors for repair
- Transfer heat to other tissues

Clotting of Blood

The ability of the blood to clot is a complex, balanced physiological process involving blood platelets, and up to 12 different clotting factors found in the blood plasma including calcium.

This is often referred to as *haemostasis* which describes the balanced process whereby damaged blood vessels are repaired to minimise blood loss, yet the clot is limited to the point of injury to maintain blood in a fluid state.

The ability for clot production inside a vein has a special interest in phlebotomy in that it is one of the factors which dictates the order that tubes are filled. This is referred to as the *'Order of Draw'* and is discussed in more detail in Chapter 8.

The blood clotting process is time related. Therefore, if a sample is required for clotting analysis, it is important that the sample is taken before a clot has time to develop. Once blood is in the clotting tube, it mixes with citrate, which binds calcium necessary for blood clot formation (Factor IV) thus preventing the clotting process from completing. In Figure 7, a schematic representation of clot formation within a vein during phlebotomy is shown and illustrates why samples for clotting analysis are amongst the first to be filled.

Figure 7 explanatory text

1. The tourniquet is applied, to distend the vein but also causes venous stasis. The needle has penetrated the vein wall and a small amount of damage has occurred to the cells which line the wall of the vein.

2. The damaged endothelial cells release a substance called *Tissue factor* in response to injury and collagen fibres in the sub-endothelial layer are exposed. *(See also Figure 16).*

3. Tissue factor causes platelets to aggregate near the area of damage. They change shape, and attach themselves to the exposed collagen fibres via Von Willibrands factor.

4. Tissue factor triggers the clotting cascade where up to 12 different components including calcium form a protein strand called *fibrin* which binds to the damaged area trapping platelets and other blood cells forming a dense plug over the damaged area.

5. If the coagulation sample tube is filled last, clotting factors, fibrin and micro-clots may be collected into the tube invalidating the results.

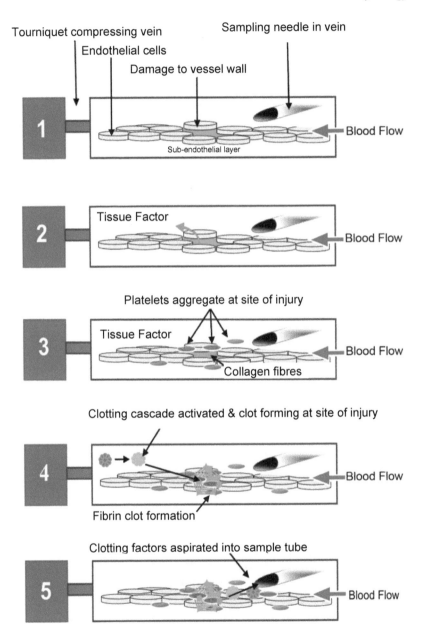

Figure 7. Schematic representation of blood clotting within a vein during sampling. (See explanatory text).

Table 1. Clotting Factors

I	Fibrinogen	VIII	Anti-Haemophiliac
II	Prothrombin	IX	Christmas Factor
III	Tissue Factor	X	Stuart-Prower
IV	Calcium	XI	Prothrombin antecedent
V	Proaccelerin	XII	Hageman factor
VII	Proconvertin	XIII	Fibrin Stabilising factor

Blood Grouping Systems

Blood grouping is attributable to the work of Karl Landsteiner (1868 – 1943) an Austrian immunologist and pathologist who discovered the ABO blood grouping system while working at the Vienna Pathological Institute.

Landsteiner discovered basic differences in blood which explained the dangers previously encountered in transfusing blood from one person to another. In 1900 he described three blood types, which he named A, B and O.

A year later in 1901, he discovered a fourth group, AB and was awarded the 1930 Nobel Prize in Physiology or Medicine.

Landsteiner with Alexander Wiener and Philip Levine discovered the Rhesus factor (Rh) in 1940.

The ABO Grouping System

Red Blood Cells

The patient's blood group will depend on the presence or absence of two antigens on the red cell surface membrane. These antigens are known as A and B.

Red blood cells in Group A have the A antigen on their surface membrane while red blood cells of Group B have the B antigen. Blood Group AB have both A and B surface antigens whilst blood Group O has neither A nor B. (See Figure 8.)

Blood Plasma

The blood plasma of an individual of blood Group A carries an antibody directed at blood Group B. Those with blood Group B have an antibody directed at destroying blood Group A. Individuals with blood Group O carry both A & B antibodies while those of blood Group AB carry neither.

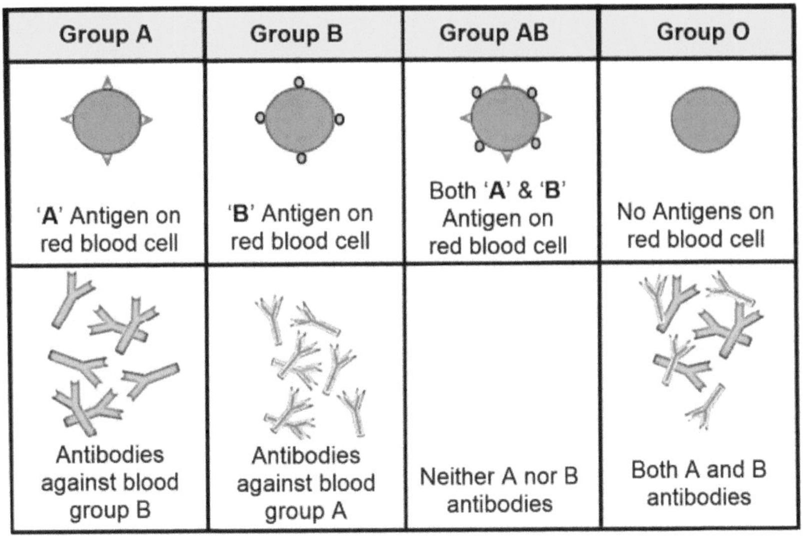

Group A	Group B	Group AB	Group O
'A' Antigen on red blood cell	'B' Antigen on red blood cell	Both 'A' & 'B' Antigen on red blood cell	No Antigens on red blood cell
Antibodies against blood group B	Antibodies against blood group A	Neither A nor B antibodies	Both A and B antibodies

Figure 8. Diagram showing surface antigens on red blood cells and antibodies in the plasma.

There are many other antigens on the surface of the red blood cells representing separate blood grouping systems such as Kell, Duffy, Lewis and Kidd but the ABO system is the most important in terms of blood transfusion.

In the event of an incompatible blood transfusion, the patient may rapidly collapse and die: less than 10 millilitres (ml) of incompatible blood can cause an anaphylactic reaction resulting in the patient's death. If this is prevented by medical intervention, antibodies bind to the antigens on the corresponding red blood cells causing the cells to agglutinate (Figures 9 & 10).

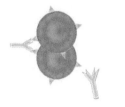

Figure 9. Antibodies bind to red blood cell surface antigens.

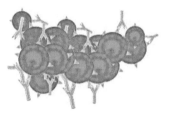

Figure 10. Red blood cells clump together (agglutination). These clumps of cells collect in the kidneys and lungs.

The clumps of agglutinated cells become trapped in the capillaries of the alveoli of the lung and or lodged in the kidneys. The tissue surrounding these clumps of agglutinated red cells become deprived of blood and oxygen, and as a result, die. The tissue cells will eventually be replaced by scar tissue but this can never act like the normal organ cells. Consequently, a patient surviving an incompatible blood transfusion can be left with severe and chronic kidney or lung disease.

Dangers of an Incompatible ABO Transfusion

◆ Death
◆ Chronic Kidney Disease
◆ Chronic Lung Disease

Figure 11. Agglutinated cells are eventually broken up.

Therefore the role and responsibility of the phlebotomist is enormous and any mix up of patients or samples can have devastating consequences.

Eventually, the clumps of agglutinated red blood cells are broken up by the body for removal. This process releases the red pigment (haem) which causes the patient to become jaundiced.

The Rhesus Blood Grouping System

This is the second most important blood group system where again the red blood cells carry the Rhesus antigen. There are several genes involved but the one which confers Rhesus Positive blood is called the D antigen. For this reason patients are said to be Rhesus (Rh) D positive or Rh D negative.

This system is especially important to young women who are of child bearing age as an incompatible transfusion can prime their immune system to produce Rh D Positive antibodies.

If the mother to be is Rh D Negative, and the father is Rh D Positive, the foetus will be Rh D Positive as the D Positive is the dominant gene. Should the patient be inadvertently transfused with incompatible Rhesus blood, or if during labour, some of the baby's blood enters the mother's circulation, she may go on to produce Rh D antibodies. During a second or subsequent pregnancy, these antibodies will destroy the developing Rh D Positive foetal blood cells leading to a condition known as Congenital Haemolysis of the New-born or 'Blue baby syndrome'.

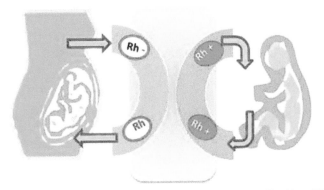

Figure 12. Mother is Rh D Negative; the foetus is Rh D Positive. Blood circulates through the placenta without any problems.

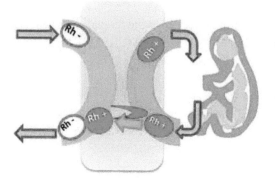

Figure 13.
At delivery, haemorrhage causes some of baby's blood to enter mother's circulation.

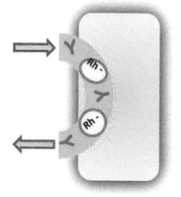

Figure 14. Mother's immune system produces Rh D antibodies in response.

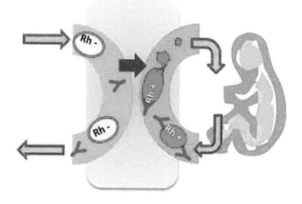

Figure 15. At the next pregnancy, the mother's blood carries the Rh D antibody which destroys the foetal red blood cells leading to congenital haemolysis of the new-born or 'Blue baby syndrome'.

Usually at the time of the first pregnancy, Rhesus Negative mothers are given Anti–D to prevent Rh D Positive antibodies from forming. However, in the case of an incompatible rhesus transfusion, the immune system becomes primed with Rh D Positive Antibodies. This can present enormous problems to young women who wish to conceive.

This section has attempted to show the potential dangers to patients of an incompatible transfusion and why it is so important that the sample is matched to the patient. Wrong Blood In Tube incidents discussed in the last chapter are the responsibility of all staff who undertake phlebotomy. As the incidence has risen over the last four years, there clearly remains a great deal of work to do in terms of training and ensuring that all staff who undertake phlebotomy are competency assessed and given the status they rightly deserve.

◆ Always check the patient's identity
◆ Label tubes at the bedside from the ID Band
◆ Never use pre-labelled sample tubes
◆ Never exceed your level of experience
◆ If in doubt, discard the sample and obtain a fresh one.

Blood is a living, liquid tissue. A Blood Transfusion is a liquid transplant.

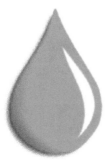

Phlebotomy must be a liquid biopsy...

References & Further Reading

1.   Pallister C.J. Biomedical Sciences Explained - Haematology.
     1999. 2-4. 65-67. Butterworth-Heinemann. Oxford.

2.   Overfield J, Dawson M, Hamer D, Pallister CJ [editor] Biomedical
     Science Explained – Transfusion Science. 1999. Butterworth-
     Heinemann. Oxford.

3.   Martini F, Ober C [et al]. Fundamentals of anatomy &
     physiology. 5th Ed. 2001. 635-639. Prentice Hall. New Jersey.

ANATOMY

6

The circulatory or vascular system consists of the heart and blood vessels arranged as a continuous closed loop system. Arteries carry oxygenated blood away from the heart into smaller arteries called arterioles, and then into capillaries which lie within the tissues. Their walls are single cell thick allowing for diffusion of water, oxygen and nutrients and collection of cell waste and carbon dioxide from metabolic processes. On leaving the capillary beds, deoxygenated blood flows into small veins called venules, eventually forming the larger veins.

Veins in the lower extremities and the arms have numerous one-way valves. Their role is to assist the low pressure venous blood return by preventing back flow caused by gravity.

Both veins and arteries are comprised of three main layers–

Tunica intima – or inner lining is composed of thin, flat cells that are arranged like paving slabs to provide a smooth inner surface which is continuous throughout the circulatory system – including the lining of the heart. These cells are also known collectively as *endothelium* and form *endothelial tissue*.

Tunica media – in veins this is a thin muscle layer but in arteries this is much thicker to resist the high arterial pressure and allows the artery to expand with the pulse.

Tunica adventitia – this a tough fibrous coat which gives support and attaches the vein to the surrounding tissues to help anchor it in position.

Nerve supply

Both veins and arteries are controlled by nerves from the *autonomic nervous system* which regulates the diameter of the vessels thereby controlling the amount of blood circulating to a particular part of the body at any one time. For example, in warm climates, veins near the surface of the skin dilate to increase blood flow allowing blood to lose heat through the skins surface whilst in colder climates, the peripheral circulation closes down to direct heat to the main body organs.

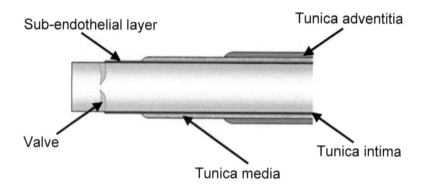

Figure 16. Diagram of a vein showing tunica layers, sub-endothelial layer and valve.

Difference between veins and arteries

Veins
Return darker deoxygenated blood back to the heart
Have a thin muscular wall
Low pressure
Contain valves
Do not pulsate
Located nearer to the surface of arms and hands
Feel soft and springy

Arteries
Carry bright red oxygenated blood from the heart to the body tissues
Thicker muscular wall
High pressure
Do not have valves
Located more deeply
Arteries pulsate

Beneath the surface of the endothelial cells, lies the sub-endothelial layer. This has an important function in aiding blood clotting in times of injury or for example after a blood sample has been taken. (*See Chapter 5.*)

Veins of the Arm

The area in the bend of the arm is the most used in phlebotomy because invariably, there is a choice of veins which tend to be located near the surface. Even in quite large individuals, the veins here can be reasonably prominent as fatty tissue tends not to be deposited where there is compression which naturally occurs at the bend of the elbow through day-to-day activity.

Veins Suitable for Phlebotomy

Everyone has slightly different anatomical features such as facial features, and body shape. This is equally true when it comes to the position of veins, arteries and nerves in the arms. From the diagram (Figure 17) it can be seen that in the bend of the elbow – often called the antecubital fossa - there are potentially four veins which could be used for phlebotomy. On some patients, there may only be one or two veins which can be seen or felt. Therefore, when choosing a puncture site, the phlebotomist invariably has little alternative but to go for the most prominent vein. Always select large surface veins which are visible or easily palpated.

The Main Veins Used are –

The Median Cubital – often this vein is larger than the median cephalic and runs nearer the surface of the skin. It is also known as the *Median Basilic vein*. Pain nerve endings appear to be less pronounced in the cubital area of the arm making the procedure less painful for the patient. However, care must be taken to avoid the brachial artery by palpating the vein to ensure it is non-pulsatile. The brachial artery should run deeper at this point but it is possible to find subsidiary arteries running nearer the surface.

The Median Cephalic - may be the only option in some patients and care must be taken to avoid puncture high up where underlying nerves may be damaged.

The Cephalic - this can often be palpated in muscular patients and is located on the outer side of the arm. Pain appears to be more pronounced in areas of the skin where there is hair growth but usually there are no underlying structures such as nerves or arteries.

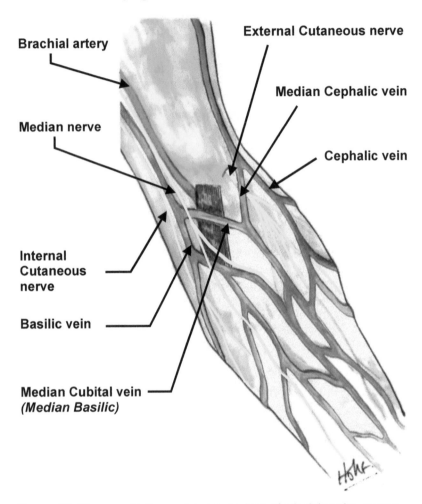

Figure 17. Diagram of left arm showing position of principle veins, nerves and the brachial artery. Note that nerves can pass over or under the veins.

The Basilic vein – This vein is best avoided completely or at least treated as the absolutely last resort because although it may be prominent in some patients, the *Internal Cutaneous Nerve* often follows the course of the vein, sometimes alongside, sometimes running underneath, and occasionally crossing over the surface.

The *Median nerve* also follows the brachial artery making nerve damage a real possibility. The brachial artery is also running very near and in elderly and emaciated patients, the artery may be seen clearly pulsating.

When veins in the cubital area are unavailable, consider obtaining the sample from the back (dorsum) of the hand using a winged collection set.

Some Phlebotomy Departments restrict access to the dorsal veins of the hand, allowing only experienced or senior phlebotomists to use them. Always check with your supervisor and follow your Department's Policy.

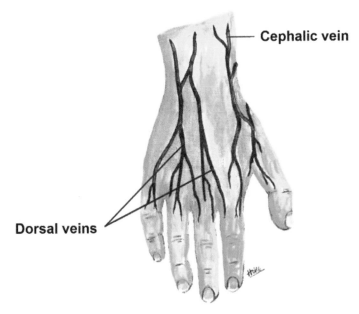

Figure 18. Diagram showing the veins on the dorsum of the hand.

Arterial Puncture

Inadvertent arterial puncture can be avoided by careful palpation of the proposed puncture site to ensure the vessel chosen is non-pulsatile. This is good practice as in cases of aberrant anatomy a subsidiary artery may lie in the space normally occupied by the vein.

If an artery is inadvertently punctured during phlebotomy, either a sudden swelling at the puncture site may appear due to the higher arterial pressure or blood flowing into the tube may appear to be a brighter red. Release the tourniquet and remove the needle and immediately apply firm pressure for at least 3 minutes. If the patient is on anticoagulants such as warfarin, this may need to be extended to 5 or 6 minutes and must be reported to the person in charge of the patient's care and documented in the patient notes. The puncture site and finger tips should be observed afterwards as the artery may go into spasm resulting in reduced blood flow to the extremities.

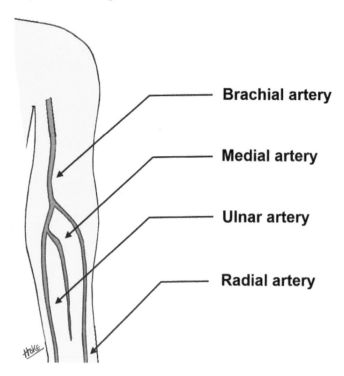

Brachial artery

Medial artery

Ulnar artery

Radial artery

Figure 19. The main arteries of the arm.

Tendons

When using the elbow, remember there is a tendon which lies centrally in the antecubital fossa area. This can be located easily by slightly flexing the elbow. The tendon will be raised and feel quite firm.

When palpating for suitable veins on the back of the hand, take care to avoid the tendons (one for each finger) which lie beneath the skin. On relaxed, chubby hands, tendons can feel like a large 'bouncy' vein. To be sure what you are feeling is a vein, move the fingers: if it is a tendon it will move with the corresponding finger.

Nerves

The main nerves in the antecubital area are –

Internal Cutaneous Nerve

This nerve is located on the inner side of the brachial artery and divides into an anterior and a posterior branch.

The anterior branch is the larger of the two and *usually* passes in front of the *Median Cubital vein* but sometimes it is behind. It descends anteriorly on the ulnar side of the forearm.

The posterior branch passes downwards on the inner side of the basilic vein to the back of the forearm towards the wrist.

External Cutaneous Nerve

This nerve often presents frequent irregularities. Usually, it emerges as a cutaneous branch slightly above the bend of the elbow and passes behind the *Median cephalic vein*. It divides at the elbow joint into an anterior and posterior branch.

The anterior portion descends along the radial side of the forearm towards the wrist whilst the posterior branch descends along the posterior side of the radius to the wrist joint. It is suggested that this nerve descends deeply along the cephalic vein in 97 % of studies carried out by Mikuni *et al* (2013).

The Median Nerve

This nerve is so named because of the position it takes in the forearm. It runs along the inner side of the brachial artery to the bend of the elbow where it crosses obliquely towards the midline. In studies by Mikuni (2013) it was found to descend superficially along the basilic vein in 73% of cases. It is this nerve which gets 'trapped' in *Carpel tunnel syndrome.*

Mikuni and co-workers suggest that the area from the middle segment of the Median cubital vein to the join with the median cephalic appears to be a relatively safe venepuncture site. These findings are supported by cadaveric dissections (Yamada *et al* 2008). Whilst they state that the distribution of cutaneous nerves varies widely and that there is no single area suitable for all individuals, they also suggest that venepuncture of the median cubital vein near to the median cephalic vein is the area least likely to cause nerve damage.

Nerve Injuries

Nerve injuries fortunately, are rare but phlebotomy is a medical procedure and, no matter how simple or minor, there is always a risk. The Phlebotomists task is to eliminate risk wherever possible by choosing safe access sites and good technique.

Sometimes nerve injury is transient and leaves no lasting affects but occasionally, patients can experience pain for many months or injury may be permanent with some loss of function. Where this occurs litigation is likely with the patient suing for clinical negligence.

For this reason, every phlebotomist should be able to name the veins in the cubital area and describe the usual location of nerves, tendons and arteries. It is not enough to simply insert a needle into the arm. Phlebotomists should know what the risks are and what to do to guard against them. Put simply, if you know the risks and actively guard against them, you cannot be negligent.

Because each one of us is different anatomically, there is always the chance of aberrant anatomy - where someone has a nerve or an artery where it would not normally be found or where it is found in a minority. We can do little about that and there is no way the phlebotomist can know where an aberrant nerve is running and there is no simple test they could perform to elicit an abnormality.

If the phlebotomy needle were to touch a nerve, the patient may complain of severe pain at the site or electric 'shooting pain' travelling up or down their arm – even to the finger tips. Remove the tourniquet and withdraw the needle. The incident should be reported to the person in charge and documented in the patient's notes stating which vein was used.

In the event of an untoward event –

◆ **Release tourniquet**

◆ **Remove Needle and dispose**

◆ **Apply dressing to puncture site**

◆ **Reassure patient**

◆ **Seek advice from supervisor**

◆ **Ensure Adverse Incident Report is completed.**

Remember, if you have no documentation, you have no defence.

References & Further Reading

1. Mikuni Y, Chiba S, Tonosaki Y. Topographical anatomy of superficial veins, cutaneous nerves, and arteries at venepuncture sites in the cubital fossa. *Anatomical Science International.* Jan 2013; 88(1): p46-57. Accessed January 2015.

2. Yamada K, Yamada K, Katsuda I, Hida T. Cubital fossa venipuncture sites based on anatomical variations and relationships of cutaneous veins and nerves. *Clin Anat.* May 2008; 21(4): p307-13. Accessed January 2015.

3. Gray H. (Edited by Pickering Pick T, Howden R). Anatomy, Descriptive and Surgical. Revised from 15th Edition. Galley Press. Leicester.

EQUIPMENT

7

One of the most basic considerations for phlebotomy is the work area. When working on hospital wards, the phlebotomy trolley becomes the workstation – carrying everything from needles and sample tubes to bar-code scanners and the environment varies from patient to patient and ward to ward. Some patients may be in bed while others may be sat out in an easy chair. In other instances, the patient is surrounded by drip-stands and infusion pumps making access to the bedside difficult with the result that the phlebotomy trolley is too far from the patient to be accessible if additional tubes are required.

In these situations, all the materials needed to obtain the sample should be placed in a clean tray or receiver and taken to the bedside. When patients are seated in an easy chair, a pillow can be placed under the patient's arm to provide comfort and support. To prevent cross infection, re-useable trays must be cleaned after each patient use. Where available, disposable cardboard trays are preferable.

When working in phlebotomy clinics, the room should be well stocked and items arranged so that everything required is to hand and within easy reach.

Most GP surgeries use the Treatment Room which contains standard chairs or an examination couch. The latter is useful for patients who have a history of fainting and any patient who reports previous faints should be asked to lie down.

The Phlebotomy Chair

A specially designed and built phlebotomy chair despite its usefulness is often considered a luxury in most areas except Phlebotomy Departments. These chairs have adjustable arm rests on both sides and have a quick release mechanism to flatten and tilt the chair to a head down position should the patient faint.

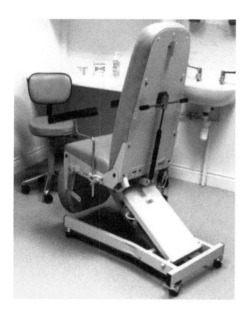

Figure 20. A phlebotomy chair with double armrests. Behind the chair is a release mechanism to lower the back down if the patient feels unwell. Note the mobile stool with backrest.

The Ideal Phlebotomy Room

The phlebotomy room should offer an acceptable level of privacy for the patient. It should be bright and well lit with natural daylight and or daylight fluorescent tubes. It should be maintained at a comfortable temperature which does not fluctuate with the seasons.

It must have adequate hand washing facilities and have a suitable work-surface which is easy to clean and on which the phlebotomist can place equipment and request forms and facilities for storage of supplies. There should also be an ergonomically designed stool for the phlebotomist to prevent back injury through repeatedly bending low over patients' arms.

The phlebotomy chair should be so arranged that access to a work surface exists on either side of the patient if fixed or a small moveable trolley should be available so that any additional items can be reached during the procedure in the event an item such as a blood collection tube is dropped on the floor.

Sharps containers should be to hand, preferably on a stand with castors so that the container can be easily and safely moved to either side of the patient. The containers should be secure so that they cannot be knocked over and stored out of reach of small children who, by necessity, may have to accompany their mothers who are having a blood test.

Access should be sufficient to permit patients using walking frames or in wheelchairs to do so comfortably. There should also be a coat peg so that patients having to remove outer clothing can at least hang their coat up.

A call button should also be provided so that the phlebotomist can summon assistance if required.

Periodically, a risk assessment should be carried out to assess the suitability of the room and its fixtures and fittings for both patients and staff members alike.

In departments where paediatric phlebotomy is carried out, the waiting area should be child friendly and have a suitable activity area.

Tourniquets

Traditionally, a tourniquet is part of the phlebotomist's apparatus and used to impede blood flow so that the veins are distended to facilitate venepuncture. Many practices are now using the single-use disposable type tourniquet ranging from special paper types to non- latex rubber ones. Some use ingenious fastenings to facilitate quick application and easy release. Despite the current trend to use disposable tourniquets, there continues to be many re-useable tourniquets in daily use in General Practices and Health Centres.

However, a great deal of evidence to support the concept of single use tourniquets has been accumulated over the years.

It has been suggested (Leitch *et al*) that contamination of re-useable tourniquets can spread infection. Their findings indicated that this spread of infection was not so much due to bacteria on the patients skin but from the phlebotomists' hands. Re-useable tourniquets are handled frequently from patient to patient and (unless there is a strict cleaning regime), from one week to the next.

Figure 21. The 'Saint' tourniquet (Sinia Medical) uses a simple quick fastening method. Also available in paediatric Size. (Available through Greiner).

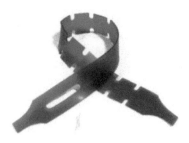

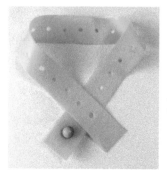

Figure 22. The Vygon Vene-K tourniquet. Application and removal is by the simple stud fixing.

In a further study (Rourke *et* al) a sample of 200 tourniquets from health professionals working in a large teaching hospital revealed 37.5% (75) had visible blood stains – with laboratory phlebotomists accounting for 69.2% and junior hospital doctors 72.7%. This is important as blood is the carrier of blood-borne infections such as HIV and hepatitis B and C. They also noted that tourniquets were owned on average for 1.86 years – only being replaced when the tourniquet was lost.

However, perhaps the most overwhelming evidence for using disposable tourniquets was published by Golder *et al* in The Lancet in 2000. They collected 77 tourniquets from a London teaching hospital and two large district general hospitals dividing them into one group of 50 and another of 27. The tourniquets were obtained from a variety of wards and specialist units.

They reported finding 50% of the tourniquets from the first group to be blood-stained and contaminated with a substantial reservoir of potentially pathogenic bacteria. All were heavily contaminated by skin flora including Staphylococci, Micrococci, Acinetobacter and Coryniform bacteria.

More serious pathogenic bacteria were cultured from 17 of the 50 tourniquets including the presence of E. coli, Staphylococcus aureus, Enterococcus faecalis and Stenotrophomonas.

The group of 27 was examined for contamination with HIV and Hepatitis B. Although neither of these viruses were isolated, the authors maintain that there remains a potential risk of viral transmission from tourniquets to patients and staff through broken skin such as cuts, abrasions and eczema.

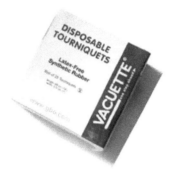

Figure 23. Simple latex free single use disposable tourniquet from Greiner Bio-One (Vacuette).

This is perfectly feasible when one considers that blood on a tourniquet is wet at the time of its attachment and could easily be transferred from one patient to another – especially in busy clinics or when treating patients who are immuno-compromised or critically ill.

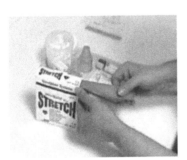

Figure 24. Simple latex-free tourniquet from Becton Dickinson (BD).

The main point of this is that as healthcare staff, we are vaccinated against Hepatitis B – most of our patients are not and therefore are the most vulnerable. Healthcare staff are advised to wear gloves to protect themselves from contact with blood and body fluids and in view of the evidence, failure to provide equal protection to patients is more than just negligent: it is to treat them as second class citizens.

Each of the studies mentioned also stress that much of the contamination arises as a result of poor hand hygiene.

Many staff members however, dislike the simple latex-free rubber strip tourniquets such as those from BD and Greiner and provide all sorts of reason why - such as they can pinch the skin and pull on hairs on the arm or they cannot be applied tight enough. They are however, incredibly comfortable for the patient, inexpensive and very easy to apply once you know how. Full details of application are shown in Chapter 11.

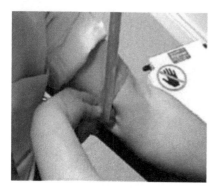

Figure 25. Applying simple strip tourniquets are easy once the technique has been acquired.

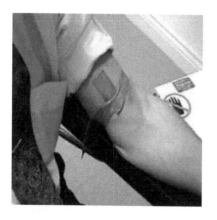

Figure 26. The tourniquet should sit flat on the arm with the ends like 'ears' protruding at the top.

The maximum time for the tourniquet to be applied is ONE MINUTE.

Multi-Sample Needles and Holders

Routine blood samples should be taken with vacuum tube devices such as those by Becton Dickinson (Vacutainer ™) Greiner Bio-One (Vacuette™), Kima (Vacutest) or the variable vacuum tubes by

Sarstedt (S-Monovette) rather than conventional syringes and needles. The S-Monovette is discussed in more detail later.

Sample tubes are pre-vacuumed so that only the correct amount of blood is taken and a multi-sample needle and holder are used.

The needle as shown (Fig. 27) is constructed of a single thin metal tube with a plastic screw-thread attachment located in the centre. The needle point is sharpened to provide a bevel cutting edge so that it cuts through the skin and into the vein. At the other end is a rubber cap which seals off the needle, preventing blood loss when attaching or removing sample tubes.

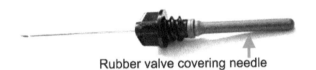

Rubber valve covering needle

Figure 27. A 22 gauge multi-sample phlebotomy needle.

To comply with the *Health and Safety (Sharp Instruments in Healthcare) Regulations 2013* needles are now provided with a safety guard either attached directly to the needle or the holder where the needle and holder are pre-assembled. These guards are designed to be operated either with the thumb or using a hard surface to swivel the guard over the needle which then locks to prevent needle- stick injury.

The Vacuette Quickshield 360™ has the needle guard attached to the holder by a ring. This allows the guard to be easily rotated and positioned on either side of the needle thereby accommodating left or right handed phlebotomists.

Needles are sized by gauge (G) and their colour coded sheaths. For example - Green, 21G and Black, 22G. The smaller the gauge number, the larger the needle. There may be a preference for using a particular needle size in your department but it makes no difference to the sample quality. This is reinforced by the work of Lippi *et al* (2006) whose investigation showed that even with finer 23G needles, such as those in winged collection sets, if handled correctly, they do not introduce any statistically or clinically significant error to the laboratory results when compared to a 21 G needle.

For preference when only one or two tubes are required, a 22G needle - being finer, causes less pain on entry through the skin and with proper skill leaves no bruising. In smaller veins, blood can bypass the needle more easily preventing the vein from collapsing.

Finer needles of course have a smaller lumen and therefore tubes take a little longer to fill. However, faced with a patient who is particularly anxious and unlikely to sit still for very long and a whole array of tubes to fill, it is conceded that a 21G may well be the better choice.

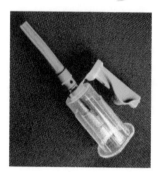

Figure 28. The Vacuette™ 'Quickshield' pre-assembled 21G needle and holder.

Figure 29. A 22 gauge 'Eclipse' needle and holder from BD. The guard is attached to the needle.

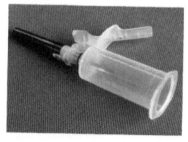

Needles are also available in 'flashback' versions by most leading manufacturers such as BD and Greiner who call theirs 'Visio plus'. On entry into the vein, blood flows back into a small see-through chamber confirming entry.

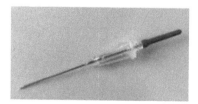

Figure 30. BD 'Flashback' needle. On entry into the vein, blood flows into the clear plastic chamber providing visual confirmation.

A description of needles and holders would not be complete with a worthy mention of the Sarstedt 'S-Monovette' system. This rather clever system looks and handles very much like a conventional syringe and needle except that the 'syringe' is in fact the sample tube. It also has the advantage that the syringe plunger can be pulled back to the lock position to pre-vacuum the tube so that the device functions just like other vacuum systems.

There are some definite advantages to this method as it allows blood to be gently aspirated into the tube. Lippi *et al* (2013) concluded that there is less chance of micro-haemolysis occurring especially when performing a difficult venepuncture combined with the negative pressure of a pre-vacuumed tube.

During difficult draws, where the blood flow is extremely sluggish, the S-Monovette system allows blood to be gently aspirated into the tube.

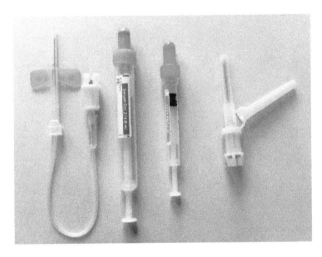

Figure 31. The S-Monovette system by Sarstedt.

Although looking very much like a syringe and needle, it is in fact a variable vacuum sample tube.

Other useful features are that once the tube is pushed onto the needle holder, a quarter turn of the tube locks it in position avoiding tubes being pushed off the needle as they fill. There is also a reduction in clinical waste as only the needle and integral mini holder go into the sharps bin because of course the syringe-type tube goes to the laboratory.

Overall, this is an excellent system, providing the usual range of needle sizes, luer adaptors and winged collection sets. The system could quite possibly eliminate haemolysis in a great many samples especially those drawn with syringes through intravenous cannulae in Emergency Departments.

Another ingenious safety device is the Greiner 'Premium' combined safety needle and holder. Attaching the sample tube activates the safety guard which automatically covers the needle on removal from the patient.

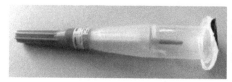

Figure 32. The Greiner Bio-One 'Premium' combined safety needle and holder.

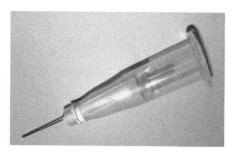

Figure 33. Inserting a sample tube activates the safety guard which rests on the skin until removal from the patient.

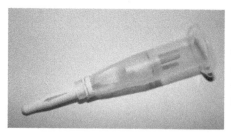

Figure 34. Removal of the device from the patient allows the safety guard to completely encase the needle thereby eliminating any possibility of a sharps injury.

Luer Adaptors

These adaptors are particularly useful for medical and nursing staff when obtaining samples from an intravenous cannula. Blood samples should only be taken at the time of initial insertion. Once the cannula has been flushed with saline it should not be used further for blood sample collection. Additionally, using cannulae for obtaining samples can cause thrombophlebitis and reduce the useful lifespan of the cannula. Always follow the hospital's Intravenous Therapy Policy or speak to the IV Therapy Team.

Other innovative equipment includes the Greiner 'Holdex' tube holder which has an off-set luer adaptor. Drawing blood through cannulae and indwelling lines is apt to cause spurious haemolysis. The Holdex is said to reduce damage to red blood cells when samples are obtained by this route - Lippi *et al* (2013).

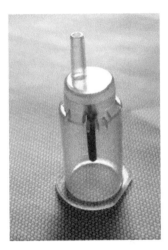

Figure 35. The 'Holdex™' needle holder by Greiner (Vacuette). The device has an offset luer adaptor and is the ideal alternative when syringe and needle techniques are used.

Luer adaptors are also used for attachment to winged collection sets and other luer fittings such as hypodermic needles or intravenous cannulae.

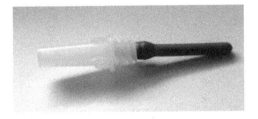

Figure 36. A luer adaptor.

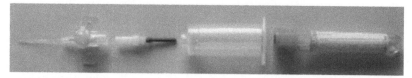

Figure 37. Exploded view of luer adaptor and an intravenous cannula. Suitable only when the cannula is first inserted.

Winged Collection Sets
Winged sets are useful for small fragile veins, when obtaining blood cultures and whenever blood samples are to be obtained from the back of the hand. All those illustrated have a safety feature and it is important that staff understand the principles of operation.

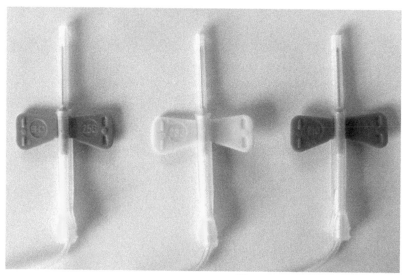

Figure 38. BD 25G, 23G and 21G Safety-Lok ™ Winged blood collection sets.

The Safety-Lok™ from BD has a yellow needle guard which slides over the needle after use. This is easy to operate one handed by holding the tubing between the fingers to anchor the needle and pushing the guard with the thumb and index-finger towards the needle point. An audible 'click' is heard and the guard can be felt locking.

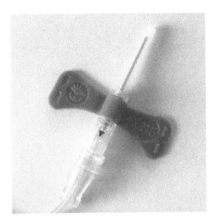

Figure 39. BD 21G self-retracting winged set. Note the small black activation button.

The self-retracting winged set from BD has a small black activation button on the clear plastic flashback chamber. When ready to remove the needle from the patient's hand or arm, the wings are stabilised, and the puncture site lightly covered with a gauze swab. Do not press on the needle or puncture site. When the black button is pressed, the spring loaded needle retracts from the puncture site and is locked into the clear plastic portion. A very clear audible click is heard.

It is wise to warn the patient that they will hear a click as the safety feature activates to avoid startling them. A colleague relayed to me her experience of an elderly lady who having heard this device click, was convinced the needle had snapped off in her arm. Seeing the device with no visible needle, only confirmed her fears.

After an identical winged set was demonstrated to her, she apparently thought they were marvellous. Patients do not appear to be the least concerned about the needle coming out—it's just the click.

The Greiner versions have a similar clear plastic chamber for the needle to retract into except this is manually operated. To remove the device, the wings are stabilised and a gauze square is placed loosely over the puncture site. At the point where the tubing joins the plastic hub, two lugs protrude. These are gently squeezed and the needle retracted from the patient's arm. Locking of the safety feature is both clearly audible and tactile.

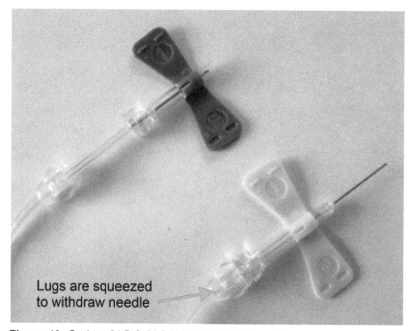

Lugs are squeezed
to withdraw needle

Figure 40. Greiner 21G & 23G Winged collection sets.

It is important that staff know how to use these safety features and are able to do so. If you are unsure, contact your line manager or ask for a demonstration from the company's representative. They should be only too happy to help.

Drawing Samples through PICC and Central Lines
Although beyond the remit of laboratory phlebotomists due to the need to administer intravenous saline flushes, medical and nursing staff may be required to draw blood samples through Peripherally Inserted Central venous Catheters (PICC) or other Venous Access Devices (VADs).

This is often the case where patients are undergoing long term chemo or antibiotic therapy and access to veins has become limited. These intravenous lines present their own problems as generally they are inserted into seriously ill patients.

The golden rule for handling any indwelling line is to perform thorough hand hygiene immediately before touching them as introducing infection could render the line unusable and most importantly, risk introducing infection directly into the central veins and in very close proximity to the heart and other major organs.

Having to remove and re-site a line not only delays treatment for the patient but may be extremely difficult to replace.

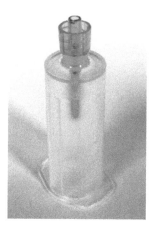

Figure 41. BD Luer-Lok adaptor for obtaining samples from indwelling venous lines.

Access to these lines always requires an aseptic technique and a trolley prepared with sterile gloves, dressing pack and sterile gauze swabs. Always follow your hospital or Trust's policy on venous access.

There are Luer-Lok devices such as the BD version illustrated which are pre-packed and sterile which can be incorporated into the procedure. The problem is that the outer surface of sample tubes are unsterile which makes performing the task aseptically difficult.

To overcome this, some practitioners hold the tube with a sterile swab or polythene bag to maintain the sterility of their glove. The swab or bag is immediately discarded afterwards. Other practitioners have little choice but to resort to a sterile syringe as the only option to maintain a totally sterile field.

Where syringes are used, a *Transfer Unit* (Fig 42) must be used to transfer the specimen into the sample tubes.

◆ Firstly, attach the syringe to the transfer unit. Gently invert the syringe and transfer unit 8 – 10 times to ensure the sample is well mixed.

◆ Holding the syringe in an upright position with the transfer unit at the bottom, attach the vacuum tubes, following the correct order of draw.

◆ Invert the tubes to mix with anticoagulant or other additive as directed.

Never remove the caps from vacuum tubes to transfer blood directly from the syringe as replacing the cap compresses the remaining air – pressurising the tube and risking blood leakage during transportation to the laboratory.

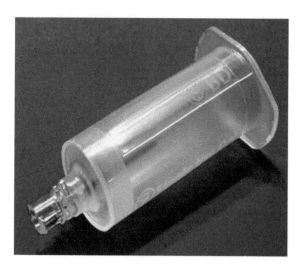

Figure 42. BD Transfer unit. This device safely transfers blood from a syringe into the blood bottle without the need for a needle to pierce the rubber stopper.

References & Further Reading

1. Leitch A, McCormick I, Gunn I, Gillespie T. Reducing the potential for phlebotomy tourniquets to act as a reservoir for methicillin-resistant Staphylococcus aureus. *J Hosp Infect.* August 2006; Vol 63: 4 p 428-431.

2. Rourke C, Bates C, Read RC. Poor hospital infection control practice in venepuncture and use of tourniquets. *J Hosp Infect. 2001; 49: p59-61.*

3. Goulder M, Chan CLH,O'Shea S, Corbett K. Potential risk of cross-infection during peripheral-venous access by contamination of tourniquets. *The Lancet.* Jan 1, 2000; 9197: p44.

8

BLOOD SAMPLE TUBES

Each laboratory speciality has its own very specific requirements for sample analysis and the requirements of one laboratory can differ to another depending on their analytical method and the equipment available to them.

Laboratories require blood specimens either as –

- Whole blood
- Plasma *(blood minus cells)*
- Serum *(blood minus cells and clotting factors)*

As a result, a wide range of sample tube types and sizes are available – each providing different properties to ensure the laboratories are presented with a suitable sample for analysis.

The examples shown here are for general guidance only and may not match your laboratory's requirements. If in doubt contact your laboratory for advice as they will have a list of tests and tube requirements.

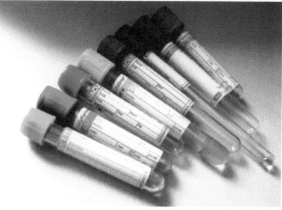

Figure 43. A selection of blood collection tubes.

Anti-Coagulant Tubes

Haematology laboratories require whole blood for full blood counts (FBC). This routine test can be used to determine a number of disorders such an infection and anaemia. In order for the laboratory analyser to count the blood cells the sample must be free from blood clots.

 This is achieved by collecting a sample in a lavender tube which has di-potassium or tri-potassium-EDTA (K2/K3-ethylene-diamine-tetra-acetic acid) which chelates or binds calcium (Factor IV) one of the coagulation factors necessary for blood clot formation. Tri-potassium EDTA may be a liquid additive whilst the di-potassium EDTA is spray coated inside the tube during manufacture which gives rise to the slightly chalky appearance to the inner tube wall.

After sample collection, it is important to gently invert the tube 6 – 8 times to mix the blood with the EDTA. Do not shake as harsh movements can damage the red blood cells.

 The pink top tube also contains spray-dried EDTA and is often used for antibody studies and blood cross- matching. EDTA preserves the structure of the blood cells. Some laboratories use the lavender tube (above) for blood bank.

 Whole blood samples for ESR (Erythrocyte Sedimentation Rate) must also remain un-clotted and Sodium Citrate 3.2% is added to this tube usually in a ratio of 1 part citrate to 4 parts blood (1:4). Citrate precipitates calcium. Care must be taken to avoid over or under filling the tube as this will alter the citrate to blood ratio and will invalidate the test.

 Similarly, a sample for coagulation studies must also remain clot free. These tubes contain liquid Sodium Citrate 3.2% as the additive. Blood in these tubes is diluted in a ratio of 1 part citrate to 9 parts blood (1:9). These tubes are used for INR, APTR and other clotting factor assays.

It is essential that these tubes are filled correctly to the indicator line marked on the tube.

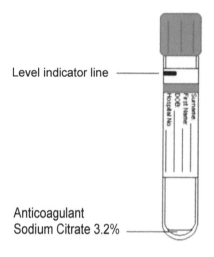

Level indicator line ————

Over or under filling will render the sample invalid and it will not be tested.

The tube should be inverted several times immediately after the sample is taken.

Anticoagulant
Sodium Citrate 3.2% ————

Figure 44. A citrate tube used for coagulation studies such as INR, APTR and APTT.

The dark green tube is used by some laboratories for chemistry tests on plasma. The additive is either sodium or lithium heparin which inhibits thrombin activation which is necessary for clot formation. Heparin is also used clinically to treat deep vein thrombosis and pulmonary embolism.

Clot Activator Tubes

Clot activator tubes promote blood coagulation, thereby removing blood cells and clotting factors leaving the serum for analysis.

Plastic blood tubes delay clotting so chemically inert activators such as silica or clay are added. This promotes clotting by providing a greater surface area for platelet attachment and activation.

The plasma portion of blood is referred to as serum once the blood has clotted and the sample centrifuged.

Serum Separator Tubes (SST)

These tubes contain a clot activator (silica) and a gel substance which separates the blood cells from the serum and are widely used in biochemistry. Once the blood has clotted - usually about 30 minutes after obtaining the sample, the tube should be centrifuged. This rapid motion causes the thixotropic gel to soften and liquefy. The density of the softened gel is less than that of the blood cells and so it rises above the level of the cells forming a barrier between the cells and serum. Once left to stand, the gel re-solidifies forming a tight seal between the cells and serum.

 Separation is necessary as most of the body's potassium is inside the cells. If separation is delayed, potassium leeches out of the red blood cells causing an increase in the serum level leading to erroneous results. Prolonged delay in commencing centrifugation will also invalidate phosphate and glucose as much of the latter will have been metabolised by the blood cells in the sample.

Once samples are taken they should be kept at room temperature 20 – 25°C and away from direct sunlight and heat sources and ideally they should reach the laboratory within about two and a half hours of being taken.

Do not store these tubes in a refrigerator as the cold encourages potassium to leech out of the cells, invalidating many other parameters.

Because these samples will have clotted within 30 minutes, a centrifuge is used to 'spin' the samples down to separate the serum from the cells. It is serum which the biochemistry department analyse.

The serum is also checked for signs of haemolysis - where ruptured red cells release their red pigment called *haem*. Where this is evident, the serum takes on a pale pink to red appearance depending on the degree of haemolysis that has occurred. Haemolysis invalidates many parameters as potassium is also released during this stage.

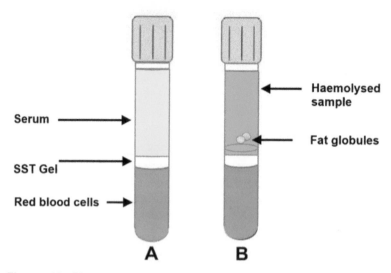

Figure 45. Diagrammatic representation of a normal sample [A] after centrifugation and a haemolysed sample [B] showing a pinkish - red tinge. Note the SST gel has risen to separate the serum from the cells. In cases of high lipidaemia, fat globules can occasionally be seen in the serum whilst in jaundiced patients the serum can take on a brownish tint.

Additive Tubes

 The grey top tube is commonly used for fasting blood glucose and the glucose tolerance test. Although glucose levels can be determined from an SST tube, glycolysis by white blood cells can deplete the glucose level substantially if there is a delay in testing. This is markedly increased where white cell counts are raised as in cases of infection.

The additives are either sodium fluoride or lithium iodoacetate which inhibit glycolysis, preserving glucose for up to 72 hours or around 24 hours for lithium iodoacetate.

To prevent clotting, potassium oxalate is added which precipitates calcium thus acting as an anticoagulant similar to EDTA.

 The royal blue tube is used for trace elements and some nutritional analysis. The additive may be either sodium heparin, Di-potassium EDTA or plain with a silica clot activator. Due to the variation in additives for this tube, to avoid confusion it has been omitted from the order of draw list.

Practitioners are advised to identify the additive in the type used in their facility and place it at the appropriate point in the order of draw. For example if it contains sodium heparin, it should be drawn after the lithium heparin, if it contains EDTA the sample should be taken with the other EDTA tubes.

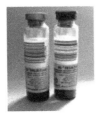 Blood culture bottles are usually supplied in pairs – one for aerobic bacteria and the other for anaerobic bacteria. The additive is tryptic soy protein which provides all the nutrients required by bacteria to survive and replicate.

Figure 46. A pair of blood culture bottles for aerobic and anaerobic bacteria.

Special precautions are required when taking blood cultures to avoid contamination and is discussed in more detail in Chapter 12.

Blood Cultures are always taken first in 'Order of Draw'.

Order of Draw
When obtaining samples there is always the risk that one additive may carry over into the next sample tube causing interference and erroneous results. A general guide is given to suit most situations but this may differ slightly from your Trust Policy which you should follow. Because not all manufacturers use the same tube colour codes, the additives are listed and the order should follow the additives.

**If in doubt, always consult your
Blood Science Laboratory.**

Order of Draw

Stopper	Additive	Indications	Inversions
	Tryptic-Soy Protein broth	Blood Cultures Ideally, 10 mls per bottle **Aerobic** then **Anaerobic**	3 - 4
	Sodium Citrate 3.2%	INR, APTR, APTT, All Coagulation screening	3 - 4
	Sodium Citrate 3.2%	ESR (Erythrocyte Sedimentation Rate)	3 - 4
	Silica	Viral serology, antibiotic levels	5
	SST gel	All biochemistry, C-RP	5
	Lithium Heparin	Plasma biochemistry Chromosomes	8 – 10
	Potassium EDTA	FBC, HbA1C, Blood Bank, ESR	8 - 10
	EDTA	Blood Bank, Antibody screen Whole blood tests	8 - 10
	Sodium Fluoride / Potassium Oxalate	Fasting Glucose, Glucose tolerance test	8 - 10

Table 2. The Order of Draw

Rationale behind Order of Draw

1. **Blood cultures** are always carried out first because of the potential for stray bacteria to enter the bottles and proliferate to the extent that the true causative organism is missed.

   The order of draw is Aerobic (Blue) then Anaerobic (Maroon). The reason is that any air within the winged collection set is sterile and will not contaminate the aerobic bottle but could prevent anaerobic bacteria replicating.

   If cultures are not required, continue with the remaining Order of Draw.

2. **Pale Blue.** Because coagulation of blood is time related, it is important to take coagulation screening samples before clotting has commenced within the vein. Samples taken later may contain micro blood clots which would affect the results.

3. **Black.** These samples are also obtained earlier in the process as micro clot formation would affect the Erythrocyte Sedimentation Rate. Essentially, the test is timing the rate red blood cells settle to the bottom of a tall narrow tube.

   If the blood cells are coated with antibodies or clumped together they will be heavier and therefore settle to the bottom of the tube more quickly. Formed micro blood-clots will also be heavier and will settle quickly producing a raised ESR – suggestive of an infection.

4. **Red Plain tubes** are taken next. They usually have silica as a clot activator. It is important that these tubes follow the citrate tubes in case the clot activator interferes with the coagulation samples. If some silica were to be carried over to the biochemistry tube it would be of no consequence because the SST sample tube invariably contains silica as a clot activator.

5. **Gold SST tubes** are taken next and because this is a clotted sample it must be obtained before any tube which contains an anticoagulant such as heparin or EDTA.

6. **Green Heparin tubes** are obtained prior to the EDTA tubes. This is to ensure potassium EDTA blood is not carried over into the heparin tube as EDTA chelates calcium which would produce a low calcium and raised potassium level in the sample. It is important that heparin tubes follow the SST tube as heparin can affect the clotting process necessary for serum samples.

7. **Purple top** EDTA tubes follow after the biochemistry SST gel tubes or green heparin plasma tubes. As stated previously, EDTA binds calcium resulting in a lower calcium level and because the EDTA additive is either di or tri- potassium EDTA, this could have a significant effect of lowering calcium and raising the potassium levels in the sample. When one considers the importance of these two substances on the heart's contractility, it becomes clear that these erroneous results must be avoided.

8. **Pink top** – EDTA tubes follow for the same reasons stated.

9. **Grey Top** – This tube is usually the last of routine samples to be drawn as the additives are potassium oxalate and sodium fluoride. Both potassium and sodium salts can interfere with electrolyte measurements in the biochemistry tubes and fluoride may inhibit a number of enzymes.

   Greiner Bio-One have produced a new sample tube (Glucomedics) which contains sodium fluoride, potassium oxalate, citrate, and EDTA to minimise glycolysis. The liquid additives will have a diluting effect on the overall results so it is important that tubes are filled to within 0.5 ml of the fill volume to ensure accuracy.

10. **Royal Blue / Other Coloured Tubes** – These tubes are used to measure trace elements such as copper, lead, mercury, selenium, zinc, arsenic, cadmium etc. They may contain sodium heparin, potassium EDTA or a serum clot activator.

    Where new or unusual tubes are to be used, always seek advice from the laboratory. Many now have their order of draw and other useful advice on their hospital or laboratory website.

HEALTH, SAFETY & HYGIENE 9

Health, safety and hygiene including infection control and prevention are essential to good practice for the patient, the phlebotomist or other practitioner, colleagues, visitors and for the hospital or employing authority.

The risks to the phlebotomist are primarily a sharps injury or contact with blood which has the potential to carry a blood-borne virus such as Hepatitis B, Hepatitis C, Hepatitis D and HIV.

In total, there are about 30 different viral infections including Cytomegalovirus (CMV), and Epstein-Barr (EBV) which can be contracted through needle-stick injury, in addition to bacterial and parasitic infections such as tuberculosis, syphilis, and malaria.

Blood Borne Virus	Potential Risk	Intervention
Hepatitis B	1:3	Post-exposure vaccine and/or Hepatitis B Immunoglobulin
Hepatitis C	1:30	Monitor risk and start early therapy in event of transmission.
HIV	1:300	Post Exposure Prophylaxis with anti-retroviral drugs.

Table 3. The possible risk of contracting a blood-borne virus from patient to healthcare worker and current intervention. Hepatitis B shows risk in unvaccinated individuals.

The potential risk figures quoted are approximations and follow a simple *Rule of Three* making the figures easier to remember. They also serve to show that Hepatitis B is statistically easier to contract than Hepatitis C or HIV.

Although the figures are approximated, there remains some disparity between the widely published figures for *potential risk* (Table 3) and those quoted for *observed surveillance* by Public Health England in their *United Kingdom Surveillance of Significant Occupational Exposures to Bloodborne Viruses in Healthcare Workers 2004 – 2013* which suggest the risks are much lower.

There are several possible explanations which collectively may have impacted on their findings. These may include current medical interventions including PEP, effective Hepatitis B immunisation; safety engineered products, products already in use, and improved risk- management. There may also have been significant under-reporting making it prudent to err on the side of caution and respect the potential risks quoted as they serve to keep us on our guard.

Immunisation

All healthcare staff should be immunised against Hepatitis B before undertaking any duties which have the potential for exposure to blood or other body fluids (WHO – *Best Practices in Phlebotomy*). Hepatitis B vaccination also protects against Hepatitis D.

Some individuals do not produce sufficient antibodies after immunisation and may be described as 'non-responders'. If you fall into this category, seek advice from your Occupational Health Department.

Sharp Injury Guidelines

You must locate and study your hospital or Trust Policy on the handling and disposal of sharps and the arrangements set up for you in the event of a needlestick injury. In some hospitals, staff attend the Accident and Emergency Department, in others they have a dedicated 'sharps' hotline.

All sharp injuries should be reported - even if they occur with a clean, sterile needle. Failure to do so reduces the risk for statistical analysis.

Where a *significant* sharps injury occurs, the staff member may be offered Post Exposure Prophylaxis (PEP) which is the anti- retroviral medication used to treat HIV. The Department of Health gold standard is that PEP should be received within an hour of sustaining injury and certainly within 24 hours. PEP is not effective after a 72 hour delay.

A 'sharps injury' is classified as *significant* if the patient is known to have (or is strongly suspected of having) one or more of these viruses. Therefore, if you receive a needle-stick injury, act immediately and follow your Trust policy.

Treatment of Needlestick Injury

◆ Gently encourage the wound to bleed.

◆ Wash the wound under warm running water using plenty of soap.

◆ **Do Not** scrub the wound while you are washing it.

◆ **Do Not** suck the wound

◆ Dry the wound and cover it with a waterproof plaster or dressing.

◆ Seek urgent medical advice from your Occupational Health Department, A & E Department or GUM Clinic.

◆ Report the injury to your employer.

◆ Complete an Incident Report.

The healthcare professional treating you will assess the risk to your health. A sample of your blood and the patient's (if known) may also be taken.

Hollow Bore Needles

Remember that phlebotomy needles have a hollow bore. The skin (and gloves) may have a 'wiping' effect on penetration – removing blood from the surface of the needle but most blood of course is held within the lumen of the needle. Withdrawal may induce a negative pressure which draws some of the blood into the tissues.

Protecting yourself

There is much that can be done to avoid both sharps injury and contact with blood and infective material.

◆ Always kept hands and fingers behind the needle.

◆ Keep sharps bin within arms-length and don't cross the sharp over your other arm to reach it.

◆ Use appropriate safety engineered devices and understand how to operate the safety features correctly.

◆ Wear enclosed–toe shoes as used needles and holders can be dropped!

◆ Wear gloves.

◆ Wear Personal Protective Equipment when required to do so.

◆ Always perform hand hygiene before applying and after removing gloves.

◆ Follow your Trust's Policies and Guidelines.

Remember, under the Health & Safety at Work Act 1974, you have a legal duty to take care of your own health and safety and that of others who may be affected by your actions. You must fully comply with measures put into place by your employer so they are able to meet their legal obligations and responsibilities.

Infection Prevention and Control

Hospitals and other healthcare settings – by their very nature - have the potential to contain an enormous range of pathogenic bacteria, viruses, fungi and parasitic organisms. To maintain our own health and well-being and to prevent the spread of infection to patients and colleagues a working knowledge of infection control is essential.

Transmission of Infection

Infectious agents can be transmitted in a number of ways –

Direct Contact – from one person to another by direct body surface to body surface contact.

Indirect Contact – this usually involves a susceptible host and an item of contaminated equipment such as a tourniquet, needles, commodes or bed rails.

Droplet Infection – Coughing and sneezing and even talking can propel small droplets of source material into the air which can carry pathogens to a susceptible host.

Airborne Infection – pathogens may be carried in the air on dust and fluff particles. Air currents can carry infectious material far from their point of origin.

Ingestion – Some infectious agents can be ingested through contaminated food and drink or through hand to mouth contact with food.

Vector Transmission – Some serious infections can be carried by other organisms which are not affected themselves. A good example of this is mosquitoes carrying malaria (*Plasmodium falciparum)* or ticks carrying Lyme disease.

The Infection Cycle

The infection cycle requires a link between three elements: pathogens, a method of transmission and a susceptible host.

Pathogens – In healthcare the initial source may be a patient or an item of contaminated equipment or a surface.

Susceptible host - Certain groups of patients such as those who have an impaired immune system will be much more susceptible than an individual who is otherwise fit and well. These patients are the most vulnerable as they have very little defence.

Transmission – This is the only area over which we can have any real influence. If we can prevent transmission, we can prevent further infection. Thorough cleaning of equipment and work surfaces reduces the number of bacteria which can be transmitted and good hand hygiene, gloves and aprons where necessary, prevent transmission to the patient.

To eliminate the risk of environmental contamination, all work surfaces and phlebotomy chairs should be cleaned with disinfectant prior to a clinic starting and whenever they become visibly soiled.

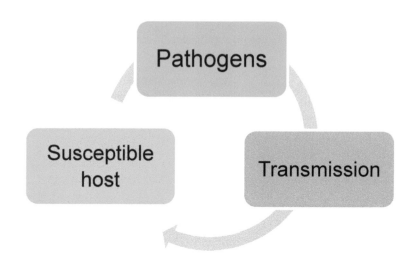

Figure 47. The Infection Cycle.

Always

- ◆ Perform adequate hand hygiene.
- ◆ Ensure all equipment and work surfaces are clean and dry.
- ◆ Ensure all sterile equipment is within date and seals are intact.
- ◆ Ensure blood spillages are cleared up using a hypochlorite solution.
- ◆ Wear Personal Protective Equipment (PPE) such as gloves and aprons as necessary.

Whenever there is a need to enter side rooms where there is a known risk of contact with infective material (Source Isolation) or when entering rooms of those patients known to have impaired immunity (Protective Isolation), PPE is essential.

Whenever there is doubt, always consult with the nurse in charge.

Hand Hygiene

One of the most effective and simplest ways of reducing the transmission of infection to our patients and ourselves is washing our hands. It has been said that hand-washing is one of the most significant things we can do for the benefit of our patients. Research has shown that the spread of infection in healthcare is largely attributed to poor hand hygiene.

The 'gold standard' is to wash hands with liquid soap and hot running water, but when this is not practicable, an alcohol hand gel may be substituted. As a guide, alcohol gel can be applied up to five times before hands need to be washed.

When to Perform Hand Hygiene

◆ On entering a clinic or hospital ward

◆ Before putting on gloves

◆ Immediately after removing gloves

◆ After contact with surfaces and objects

Always follow your Trust policy on hand hygiene.

1. Wet hands.

2. Apply liquid soap.

3. Rub palms together.

4. Rub back of both hands – fingers interlocked.

5. Rub palm to palm with fingers interlocked.

6. Rub backs of fingers (interlocked)

7. Rub thumbs in circular motion.

8. Rub both palms with finger tips.

9. Rub each wrist with a circular motion.

10. Rinse hands.

11. Turn off taps with elbows.

12. Dry hands on paper towels.

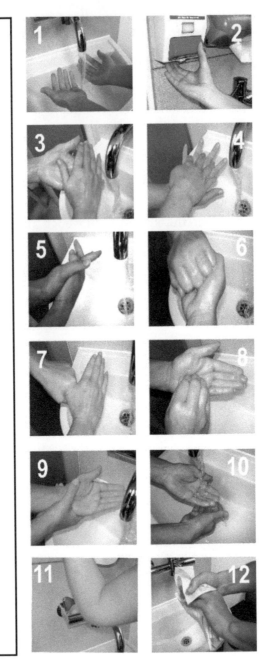

Figure 48. Hand washing sequence

Gloves

The wearing of gloves is mandatory in any situation where there is the potential to come into contact with blood or other body fluids and forms part of Standard precautions in healthcare. Gloves not only protect the healthcare worker from blood-borne viruses and other infections, they also provide protection against the transmission of infections to the patient (*WHO guidelines on drawing blood: best practices in phlebotomy*).

Gloves should not be worn when answering the telephone or using computer keyboards.

Removing Gloves, Aprons and PPE

The technique for removing gloves and aprons is important to prevent contaminating yourself with blood or bacteria. The outside of the glove must not touch your bare skin or uniform.

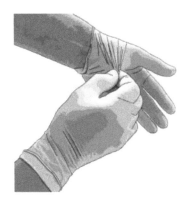

Figure 49. Grasp one glove by the palm and pull the top half of the glove over the fingers turning it partly inside out.

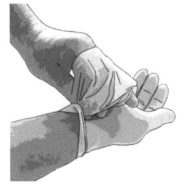

Figure 50. Grasping the second glove just above the palm, remove by pulling it inside out. Both gloves can now be handled touching only the inner side of glove 2.

Wash hands immediately after removal of gloves.

To remove contaminated gloves, grasp one glove by the palm and pull it over so that it partially covers the gloved fingers as shown in Figure 49.

Grasp the second glove with the outer side of the first glove and pull the glove completely over the fingers turning it inside out. With your now bare hand you can take hold of the inner side of both gloves and discard in the clinical waste container.

Disposable plastic aprons should be untied at the back and neck with your bare hands, not your soiled gloves. The apron should be folded in on itself folding it into a ball ensuring that you are only touching the cleaner inner side.

Discard in a clinical waste container and immediately wash your hands. This is essential as the wearing of gloves provides a warm, moist environment and as bacteria can replicate in as little as twenty minutes or less will mean there are many more bacteria on your hands when you take the gloves off than there were when you put them on.

A similar practice applies when removing face masks. Again these must be removed with your bare hands – never with your soiled gloves.

Universal Precautions

Following the emergence of HIV in the 1980's, the Centre for Disease Control and Prevention in Atlanta, USA, introduced the concept of 'Universal Precautions' which were designed to limit the spread of blood-borne viruses (BBV) to healthcare staff.

The measures were based on the premise that all blood and other bodily fluids including saliva, from any patient, may contain a BBV as many patients may of course be asymptomatic or unaware that they are infected. The concept was adopted by healthcare providers across the world.

It also had other benefits because everyone was treated as though they had a BBV, those who did, were not subjected to the humiliation where everyone wears gloves for them but not for other patients.

The Precautions included specific recommendations for use of personal protective equipment (PPE) such as gloves, protective eyewear, masks and gowns as appropriate when contact with blood, body fluids or broken skin is anticipated.

In phlebotomy, there is always the risk of coming into contact with blood or broken skin - even when applying the dressing and so for this reason, gloves must always be worn.

An equally important argument in support of wearing gloves is that just as many HIV positive patients may be asymptomatic, so too may the healthcare workers. HIV is now no longer a barrier to becoming a phlebotomist providing the viral load count is below detectable levels.

We cannot claim to be protecting patients where there is failure to implement protective measures and for patients to have confidence in the health service they must have the right to ensure they are not at risk from the healthcare professional. As mentioned previously, all healthcare workers are immunised against Hepatitis B which is 100 times more likely to cause infection than HIV yet very few of our patients are. Therefore, they are the most vulnerable. Failure to acknowledge these points can only lead to an accusation of 'double standards'.

Universal precautions were introduced by healthcare staff primarily to protect healthcare staff. However, by focusing so much on the protection of staff, we failed to adequately address the need to protect non-infected patients in our care by simple measures such using disposable tourniquets.

Standard Precautions

Standard Precautions - also known as *Standard Infection Control Precautions* are now the routine approach to reducing nosocomial or healthcare associated infections (HAI's). Standard Precautions rightly put the patient at the centre and by doing so, healthcare staff protect themselves.

Standard Precautions apply to the care of *all* patients, in *all* healthcare settings, regardless of suspected or confirmed diagnosis or presumed infective status. Implementation of Standard Precautions includes hand hygiene, and the wearing of PPE to prevent infection and cross contamination.

Therefore, to comply with Standard Precautions, hand hygiene and the wearing of gloves when performing an *exposure prone procedure* (EPP) like phlebotomy, becomes mandatory.

The terms Universal and Standard precautions are often used interchangeably to mean the same thing but they are different in their focus.

It is interesting to note that as a throwback to the Universal Precaution days, gloves and aprons are still referred to as *Personal Protective Equipment* – even when worn to protect patients. Perhaps it is time to rename them.

Many items concerning Infection Control and Health and Safety may be assessed by the Care Quality Commission (CQC) under the terms of The Health and Social Care Act 2008: *Code of Practice on the prevention and control of infections and related guidance* - January 2015.

Cleansing the Puncture Site

There remains variation in phlebotomy practice throughout the UK in terms of skin preparation. Some Trusts and Phlebotomy Departments perform skin 'prep' whilst others do not and proffer various reasons for not doing so.

Some argue that it is not necessary to prep 'visibly clean skin'. The question of course is what is their definition of 'clean'.

The purpose of prepping is to remove bacteria from the puncture site to prevent them being carried directly into the bloodstream via the needle and, as we cannot see bacteria with a naked eye, how can we be sure it is 'clean'? Whilst the skin may *appear* clean it could be heavily colonised with pathogenic bacteria. Phlebotomy should always be performed as an aseptic technique.

Another reason proffered is that it can remove the skins natural flora. Indeed, this may be so but it is only over a very small area and if destroying the natural flora is such a dreadful thing, why do we advocate so much hand-washing and use of alcohol rub?

The World Health Organisation (*WHO Guidelines on drawing blood: best practices in phlebotomy*), in consultation with expert opinion recommend skin cleansing with 2% Chlorhexidine gluconate in 70%

isopropyl alcohol, ensuring the skin area is in contact with the disinfectant for at least 30 seconds and allowed to air-dry for a further 30 seconds. Skin disinfecting products such as Steret H® or Clinell® are inexpensive and readily available through NHS Direct.

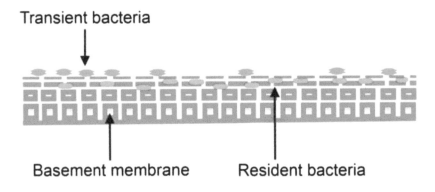

Figure 51. Diagrammatic representation of the skin showing transient and resident bacteria.

The skin consists of a basement membrane which produces skin cells. As the cells mature, they flatten and move towards the surface. Skin cells are constantly being replaced with new cells and the old ones become dry and flake off. As a result, we shed thousands of skin cells daily.

On the surface of the skin lie the ***Transient bacteria***. These are the bacteria we pick up for example on our hands and other body surfaces and which can easily be spread to patients directly or indirectly on inanimate objects that we handle.

Beneath this layer, nestled in and around the thinner, flaking skin cells lay the ***Resident bacteria***.

The material used for skin disinfecting swabs is designed to be slightly abrasive so that not only are transient bacteria removed but also dry, flaky skin cells. This exposes the resident bacteria which with proper cleansing, are also removed, leaving a relatively bacteria- free surface through which the needle can pass.

Start by cleaning at the proposed puncture site using reasonably firm pressure in an ever increasing circular motion. This aims to push bacteria and skin cell debris to the perimeter.

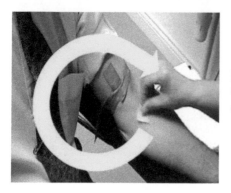

Figure 52. Skin preparation. Clean using a firm, increasing circular motion.

Do not fan, blow on, or swab the 'prepped' site to aid drying.

When performing skin cleansing on fair, pale skinned patients the swab after 30 seconds cleaning will barely show any discolouration. However, when performing this on a very dark-skinned patient, or those with a good suntan, the swab on removal can look very discoloured. Please note, this is not an indication that the patient is in any way dirty, it simply means that you have performed the skin prep effectively by removing the surface layer of dead skin cells and many of the transient and resident bacteria.

It is important that comments or distasteful facial expressions are not made as this can be extremely offensive to the patient. Even patients can be surprised at the colour of the swab so be ready to reassure the patient that it is dark skin, not dirt. If the skin is visibly dirty it should be washed first with soap and water.

Disposing of Clinical Waste
The careful and timely disposal of clinical waste is important to maintain a safe and hygienic environment. All NHS Trusts will have a policy appertaining to the disposal of waste which must be adhered to. Failure to do so can leave hospital authorities open to prosecution where it can be shown that clinical waste has found its way to landfill sites.

All sharps should be disposed of immediately after use and at the point of use. Sharps must never be carried across a ward to the sharps bin. The sharps bin must go with you and be located within easy reach.

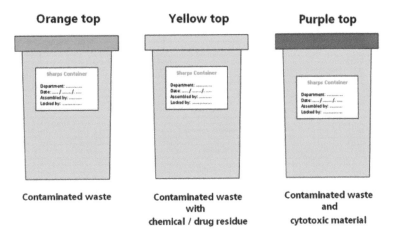

Figure 53. Sharps containers. Different coloured tops indicate their permitted contents.

Sharps containers are colour coded to indicate their contents. Those with orange tops are suitable for all phlebotomy sharps. These containers only need disinfection to destroy bacteria and blood borne viruses. This leaves the plastic and or metal components available for recycling where this is available.

The yellow top container is also suitable for phlebotomy sharps but may also contain syringes containing medication. These must be destroyed by incineration.

The Purple top container may contain cytotoxic material – residues from chemotherapy. These could contaminate waterways and pose a risk to public health so they too must be incinerated.

Sharps containers must be traceable to the person who assembled it, the person who locked it and the ward or department where it was sited. Ensure the sharps container is locked, the attached label completed and replaced when it is approximately three-quarters full.

There is an indicator line on containers to show when it is full to a safe capacity.

Never put non-sharp items such as gloves, swabs and paper in Sharps Containers: this is a costly waste of resources.

Waste disposal sacks should be attached to a foot operated stand. Never lift lids by hand. Soiled dressings and swabs must be cleared away after use and placed in the appropriate clinical waste sack – usually yellow or orange. Because of the potentially infective nature of the contents, these bags must go for incineration.

Paper hand towels and packaging may go into the general waste – usually a black bin bag and are suitable for land-fill sites.

Never allow bags to become over full so that waste material spills out onto the floor.

Law Covering Waste Disposal

Under the Environmental Protection Act 1990 it is unlawful to dispose of controlled (including clinical) waste without a waste management licence. Contravention of waste control is a criminal offence and could result in your Trust being fined thousands of pounds.

Blood spillages

All blood spillages must be treated as being potentially infectious. Minor splashes can be cleaned up using a hypochlorite solution whilst more severe spillages are usually absorbed with hypochlorite granules.

Many hospitals and NHS Trusts provide blood spillage kits which include gloves and apron, yellow or orange disposable bag with tie, hypochlorite granules, chlorine tablets and a scoop.

It is important that staff follow their Trust guidelines and policies on the correct procedure for blood spillages and clinical waste disposal.

References & Further Reading

1. Woode Owusu M, Wellington E, Rice B, Gill ON, Ncube F & contributors. Eye of the Needle United Kingdom Surveillance of Significant Occupational Exposures to Bloodborne Viruses in Healthcare Workers: data to end 2013. December 2014. Public Health England, London.

2. Health & Safety Executive. Blood-borne viruses: Available from - http://www.hse.gov.uk/biosafety/blood-borne-viruses/how-deal-exposure-incident.htm.   Accessed 16/01/2015.

3. Health & Safety Executive. Blood-borne viruses in the Workplace: Guidance for employers and employees. Available from - http://www.hse.gov.uk/pubns/indg342.pdf. Accessed 19/01/2015.

4. The World Health Organisation. WHO Guidelines on drawing blood: best practices in phlebotomy. P. xiv. http://whqlibdoc.who.int/publications/2010/9789241599221_eng .pdf   Accessed 18/03/2015.

5. World Health Organisation. WHO Standard Precautions in Healthcare. P. Xv. Available from- http://www.who.int/csr/resources/publications/EPR_AM2_E7.pdf. Accessed 21/01/2015.

6. The Management of HIV infected Healthcare Workers who perform exposure prone procedures: updated guidance, January 2014. Public Health England.

7. Department of Health. The Health and Social Care Act 2008: *Code of Practice on the prevention and control of infections and related guidance.* January 2015.

10 PRE-ANALYTICAL ERRORS

Blood samples are important in the diagnosis, treatment, and health screening of many conditions and forms one of the first steps in healthcare interventions. After the results are diligently produced by the laboratory staff and authorised, they are available for the medical and nursing staff to review.

Because there is a natural biological variation in all of us, there is no clear-cut demarcation line that differentiates between health and disease. Results are interpreted against a *Reference range* of what is 'usual' for 95% of the population.

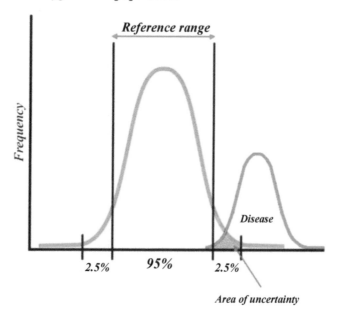

Figure 54. Graphical illustration of the Reference range in health and disease.

For example, if we were constructing a reference range for the height of men we would measure the height of a wide representative group of the male population. If we found that 95% of men were between five foot - nine inches and six foot – two inches tall, that would be our 'reference range'.

Clearly that does not include everyone - some men may be five feet – two inches while others may be six-foot – six inches tall. Their numbers are less and so they fall into the 2.5% category at each end of the distribution curve.

If we found an adult male who was six-foot nine inches tall and another male who was only four feet – six inches tall, we might consider the possibility of some abnormality – perhaps over or under production of growth hormone leading to giantism or dwarfism. However there are exceptions: some American basket-ball players can be nearly seven feet tall while Pygmies are known to be much smaller in stature. These individuals do not suffer from an abnormality; it is simply a matter of biological diversity among different populations. However, until we can establish this as fact their respective heights place them into an *area of uncertainty.*

Similarly, in terms of blood results, natural biological variations can occur as a result of-

- Gender,
- Age of the patient
- Time of day sample obtained
- Pregnancy
- Alcohol consumption
- Smoking.

Areas of Uncertainty

The importance of these 'areas of uncertainty' is that pre-analytical errors - no matter how slight and seemingly insignificant they may be on their own, compounded with other variables, they can produce very significant changes to the results. Potentially this may push the patient's results further into the 'area of disease' leading to miss-diagnosis and unnecessary treatment or alternatively pull results back into the normal reference range leading to missed diagnosis and failure to identify and treat a condition the patient does have.

It therefore falls upon all those who perform phlebotomy to be as diligent and accurate in obtaining samples as we expect the laboratory to be in analysing them. Remember, 'Inaccurate samples in - means inaccurate results out'.

Haemoconcentration

The tourniquet should never be applied for longer than one minute. If locating a suitable vein is difficult, release the tourniquet and re- apply it, keeping to the one minute time. When obtaining samples for calcium analysis, the tourniquet should not be used or the tourniquet released prior to attaching the sample tube.

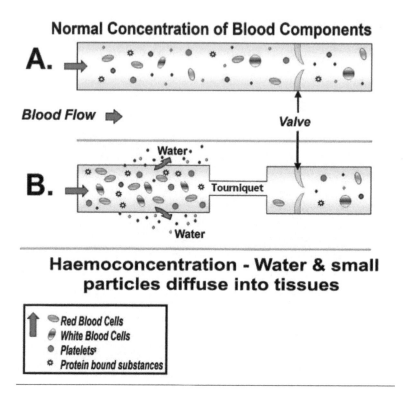

Normal Concentration of Blood Components

A.

Blood Flow ➡

Valve

B.

Water•

Tourniquet

Water

Haemoconcentration - Water & small particles diffuse into tissues

- Red Blood Cells
- White Blood Cells
- Platelets
- Protein bound substances

Figure 55. Haemoconcentration can occur through extended tourniquet times.

Haemoconcentration occurs as a result of extended tourniquet time. Venous pressure is forcing blood up the arm and, whilst the tourniquet impedes the return blood flow, it does not stop the venous pressure. The result is that water and small solutes such as potassium are able to pass through the vein and capillary walls into the surrounding tissues. Blood cells and larger components are too big to do this but as water leaves, it draws more blood and cellular components into the area increasing the concentration. The effect may be greater in patients who are hypertensive or prone to oedema.

Statistically significant clinical differences for haemoconcentration have been observed by a number of researchers. Lippi *et al* reported an increase of 1.6% in calcium after 1 minute rising to 3.6% after 3 minutes with albumin increased by 8.6% after 3 minute stasis. Other parameters such as total protein, iron, cholesterol, creatine kinase, creatinine, and glucose may also be affected. After 3 minutes of venous stasis, clinically significant results were obtained for fibrinogen, prothrombin time and D-dimers.

Another study (Burtis & Ashwood) demonstrated that when the tourniquet time is extended to 3 minutes, protein rose by 4.9%, iron by 6.7%, total lipids 4.7%, cholesterol 5.1%, Aspartate aminotransferase by 9.3% and bilirubin by 8.4%.

Just as there are several blood components which rise, there are also analytes which fall. At 3 minutes, Burtis and Ashwood found potassium decreased by 6.2%. Research by Lippi and co-workers support these findings reporting a fall in potassium of 2.8% after 1 minute and a decrease of 4.8% after 3 minutes venous stasis.

Both Potassium and calcium are extremely important to the hearts contractility and therefore active treatment on erroneous results could prove disastrous. Potassium levels are also important to patients in the pre-operative stage due to the potential interaction of muscle relaxant drugs used in anaesthesia. Surgery may need to be delayed or postponed where results are found to be outside the reference range.

Fist Clenching

Many healthcare workers, having applied a tourniquet, ask the patient to 'open and close' their fist. This should be avoided as this has the effect of raising the potassium level. A raised potassium level is called hyperkalaemia and its affect on the heart is sufficient to cause changes in an electrocardiograph (ECG). Where raised potassium is known to be false it is often termed pseudo-hyperkalaemia.

There are several explanations as to why pseudo-hyperkalaemia occurs including mechanical trauma during the venipuncture process such as harsh slapping of the vein or arm to encourage the veins to appear, fist-clenching or an excessively tight tourniquet. Slapping the arm to promote veins is unnecessary and can be painful for the patient and leave unsightly bruises.

Pseudo-hyperkalaemia in phlebotomy may be explained by considering that although the tourniquet has stopped the venous return of blood flow, the blood cells are under increasing venous pressure. Repetitive fist-clenching also causes the muscles in the forearm to add further pressure to the blood trapped by the tourniquet and the effect is that potassium is squeezed out of the blood cells into the plasma.

Additionally, it has been known since the mid-1930's (Fenn) that muscular activity can lead to additional potassium loss from the muscle cells. In 1961 Skinner demonstrated that forearm exercise could raise potassium levels and the principles were brought to light again in 1990 (Don *et al*) who produced increases of between 1 – 1.6 mmol per litre.

Considering the reference range for potassium is in the order of 3 – 5.5 mmol per litre, their results are highly significant. Additionally, there is also the analytical variable – the margin of error produced by the laboratory analysis which must be factored into the total result.

Syringe collected samples

The most reliable method for collecting blood samples is using vacuum tubes or the Monovette system. These are all 'closed' methods and offer consistency in collection.

Samples taken with a syringe are by the 'open' method and are subject to a number of variable effects especially those caused by haemolysis and blood settling in the syringe before being transferred into the sample tube.

Haemolysis can occur through harsh vacuums, especially when using 10 and 20 ml syringes and where samples are drawn through intravenous cannulae. Once lysis of the red cells occur, the cellular contents including potassium are released into the plasma which is then collected as part of the specimen. In the laboratory, haemolysis is identified by the characteristic pinkish-red colour of the serum which will invalidate the potassium level.

However, perhaps the biggest problem of all when obtaining samples with a syringe is that blood being a liquid containing cellular and other components in suspension can separate.

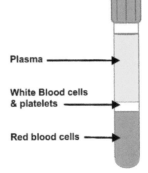

Figure 56. Blood left to stand in a sample tube separates into its component parts.

Plasma

White Blood cells & platelets

Red blood cells

Whilst blood is moving through the circulation it is well mixed. However, when left to stand – even for a short period of time, separation of the various components occur.

The larger and heaviest components such as red blood cells separate out first by sinking, followed by white blood cells and platelets which float on top. Plasma will then consist of other components arranged in layers according to their molecular weight.

The speed that this occurs, will naturally vary but can be influenced by infection and logically this will occur more rapidly in a patient whose Erythrocyte Sedimentation Rate (ESR) is high. The paradox is that the latter cannot be ascertained without a blood test.

Where there is absolutely no alternative to using a syringe, transfer to the sample tubes should be by means of a *'transfer unit'* (Figure 42.)

Once the syringe is connected, it must be gently inverted 8 – 10 times to ensure the sample is well mixed before attaching the specimen tube, following the correct order of draw.

Results should always be viewed in the light by which they were taken. Where results are unexpected, it is worth repeating the sample to eliminate any possibility of a pre-analytical error.

In the laboratory, staff are well aware of this separation and place their haematology samples on a roller which keeps the sample slowly turning over keeping it well mixed and representative of the patient's true circulating blood component levels.

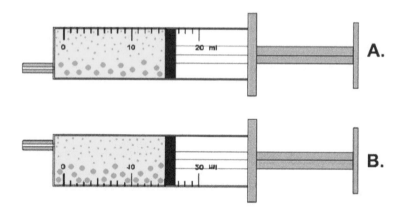

Figure 57. Diagrammatic representation showing that blood separates in a syringe resulting in uneven component transfer to the sample tube.

The above illustration (Figure. 57) shows a diagrammatic view of two syringes containing blood which have been allowed to stand for a few minutes where separation has occurred.

In (A) blood cells have settled at the base adjacent to the luer fitting. When blood from this syringe is transferred to a sample tube, (assuming it is not mixed) the red cells will enter first, raising the haemoglobin level and potentially masking a patient's anaemia.

In syringe (B) the luer fitting is at the top and when this unmixed sample is transferred into a sample tube, more plasma will enter the sample tube than blood cells suggesting the patient is anaemic, with the possibility of a higher white cell and platelet count.

To evaluate the concept of this, a series of small experiments
were conducted.

Test 1. In the following example, two phlebotomists obtained samples
simultaneously – one on the left and the other on the right arm.
Tourniquet application and release were synchronised as were the
venepuncture and tube application and removal. Samples were
analysed together in the laboratory on the same machine. Movement
of the syringe and therefore mixing of the sample was performed as
might be typical in ordinary clinical practice and the sample was
transferred to the sample tube immediately after. The results for
haemoglobin and other red cell parameters are shown in Table 4.

**Table 4. Haematology - comparison of Vacuum tube &
Syringe Samples**

	Vacuum Device	Syringe & Needle	Percent Change
Haemoglobin	14.3	15.2	+6.3
MCV	93.1	92.6	-0.5
MCH	30.9	32.5	+5.2
MCHC	33.1	35.1	+6.0
Neutrophils	5.4	5.2	-3.7

It can be seen that the largest variation occurred in the haemoglobin
analysis.

Test 2. This was obtained at the same time as the previous sample.
The results (Table 5) show that whilst there were no changes in urea
or sodium, there was a decrease of **17%** for potassium compared to the
vacuum tube control sample.

**Table 5. Biochemistry - comparison of Vacuum tube &
Syringe Samples**

	Vacuum Device	Syringe & Needle	Percent Change
Urea	5.5	5.5	
Sodium	143	143	
Potassium	**4.7**	**3.9**	**-17%**

Test 3. To evaluate how quickly blood can settle in a syringe, a 20 ml sample was obtained whilst a second phlebotomist simultaneously obtained a standard vacuum tube sample as a control.

The aim of this test was to simulate the effects of a sample taken where there is a short delay in transferring blood into the sample tube. This could easily occur when clinical staff obtain a sample perhaps in the Emergency Room when they are busy and have other matters to attend, or for example as might occur when the sample is obtained through a newly inserted intravenous cannula.

Chart 3. The effect of white cells separating out in a syringe sample.

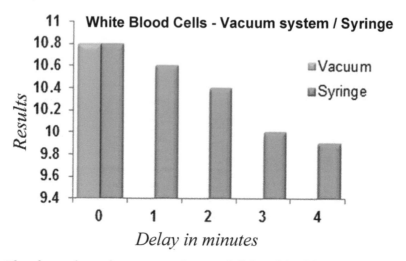

Delay in minutes

The above chart shows a continuous fall in white blood cells with the maximum decrease occurring between 2 and 3 minutes resulting in a fall of 0.4 with an overall decrease of 0.9 ($\times 10^9$/Litre) (8.3% in 4 minutes).

The reference range for white blood cells is $4 - 11$ ($\times 10^9$/Litre). Results above 11 would suggest a bacterial infection for which antibiotics may be appropriate. If the results were adjusted to show an infection, a 3 or 4 minute delay could show a normal result leading to a missed opportunity to diagnose a bacterial infection. Imagine the possibilities if this were your child with bacterial meningitis.

Over the years there have been numerous reported instances where blood having separated in a syringe has led to patients receiving inappropriate treatment such as a blood transfusion. In some instances this has led to blood having to be removed as the post-transfusion full blood count revealed alarmingly high haemoglobin levels.

In a similar case, a female patient with a haemoglobin (Hb) of 13.7 was admitted to an elderly care ward. She received daily blood tests for full blood count and urea and electrolytes. After a few days her Hb started to fall. One Saturday, the duty doctor took a syringe sample of blood and was surprised to find her Hb was 19.2 grams per decilitre. He made a diagnosis of polycythaemia (*Lit. 'Many cells'*) and contacted the Consultant Haematologist for advice – querying how much blood he should draw off to return the Hb to within the normal range of 11.5 – 15.5 g/dl.

After discussion with the Haematologist, he was advised to repeat the sample using a vacuum device and a winged needle. When the results came back the haemoglobin was 9.3 g/dl.

The elderly lady was already anaemic and drawing off perhaps 300 - 500 mls of blood would have made her even more so - perhaps needing a blood transfusion as elderly patients often take longer to replace blood loss.

Her low haemoglobin level was a result of repetitive daily blood tests which, when induced by healthcare interventions is called iatrogenic anaemia.

Remember, these principles do not apply to the S- Monovette system as this is not a syringe: it is the sample tube. Any separation with be resolved by mixing in the laboratory.

◆ Only use a syringe when there is no other choice.

◆ Ensure the sample is well mixed before transferring to a specimen tube.

◆ Always use a transfer device.

◆ Follow the order of draw.

◆ Review the results bearing in mind how the sample was taken. Repeat sample if necessary.

Reference & Further Reading

1. Lippi G, Salvagno GL, Montagnana M, Brocco G, Guidi GC. Influence of short-term venous stasis on clinical chemistry testing. *Clin Chem Lab Med*. 2005; 43 (8):869-75.

2. Burtis CA, Ashwood ER. In: *Teitz Fundamentals of Clinical Chemistry*. Fifth Edition. P32. WB Saunders.

3. Bailey IR, Thurlow VR. Is suboptimal phlebotomy technique impacting on potassium results for primary care? *Annals of Clinical Biochemistry*. May 2008; 45: 266-269.

4. Burns SD, Matchett JL. Effect of phlebotomy technique on serum bicarbonate values. *Academic Emergency Medicine*. 1998; 5. 1: 40-44.

5. Rosen RS, Tangney CC. Effects of tourniquet application on plasma viscosity measurements. *Clinical Hemorheology and Microcirculation*. 1998; 18. 2-3: 191-194.

6. Don BR, Sebastion A, Cheitlin M, Christiansen M, Schambelan M. Pseudo-hyperkalaemia caused by fist clenching during phlebotomy. *The New England Journal of Medicine*. May 3;1990: 1290-92.

7. Lippi G, Salvagno GL, Montagnana M, Guidi GC. Short-term venous stasis influences routine coagulation testing. *Blood Coagul Fibrinolysis*. 2005 Sept; 16(6): 453-8.

8. Skinner SL, Adelaide MP. A cause of erroneous potassium levels. *Lancet*. 1961; 1: p478–480.

9. Fenn WO. Electrolytes in muscle. Physiol Rev 1936; 16:450– 87.

10. Saleem S, Mani V, Chadwick MA, Creanor S, Ayling RM. A Prospective study of the causes of haemolysis during venepuncture: tourniquet time should be kept to a minimum. *Ann Clin Biochem*. 2009 May: 46 (Part 3): p 244-6.

PHLEBOTOMY TECHNIQUE 11

Before moving onto the technique, we should take a moment to briefly recap on the basic principles.

The aims and objectives of obtaining samples are to –

◆ Ensure the patient is correctly identified by open questioning and checking against ID Band (in-patient) or Request Form (out-patient).

◆ Ensure the sample is truly representative and free from artefacts. Observe the tourniquet time. No fist-clenching, tapping or slapping veins.

◆ Follow the Order of Draw to prevent additive carry-over.

◆ Ensure the sample is correctly labelled with the right patient details including four points of ID plus date, time and signature.

◆ Ensure the patient is free from bruising or haematoma.

◆ Ensure we do not spread infections to patients through poor practice. Always 'prep' the skin, wear clean gloves and PPE as required.

◆ Ensure our practice is safe by following 'Sharps Policies'.

◆ Send the sample to the laboratory in a timely manner.

◆ Seek help from a colleague or supervisor when necessary.

First Things First

On receipt of the Request Form, carefully examine it to confirm you understand the tests that are required and that you have the appropriate tubes. If the test is for a fasting sample, you will need to ask the patient when they last had anything to eat or drink. Fasting usually requires abstaining from all food and drink for 12 hours although clear water (unflavoured, non-sparkling) may be taken as required.

If the test is for therapeutic medication, you may need to note on the form when the last dose was given.

Greet the Patient

The phlebotomist or other practitioner should greet the patient and introduce themselves and state their purpose. A pleasant, confident and calm approach helps relax the patient making the task in hand easier for all concerned.

It is best not to address the patient directly by name until *they* have given their full name first. This will help identify patients who are hard of hearing or confused.

Remember, when checking the patient's identity, actively look for discrepancies not just confirmation.

Gain valid consent and be ready to answer any questions or address any concerns the patient may have. Some patients may have a needle phobia, or a history of fainting. Often, patients will be able to suggest a vein which is known to be good. It is wise to follow the patient's advice here as they know their bodies better than we do and many patients who regularly attend the clinic will have experienced and learnt from the trial and errors of past performances.

Selecting a Vein

Sometimes, for an experienced phlebotomist, suitable veins can be identified as soon as the patient sits in the phlebotomy chair. Others need more careful examination and a tourniquet may be needed at this stage to find a suitable vein.

The tourniquet should be applied approximate 4 inches (10 centimetres) above the proposed puncture site. As a general guide, this is about the breadth of a hand. Remember, the tourniquet must be removed and reapplied after one minute.

Biceps muscle

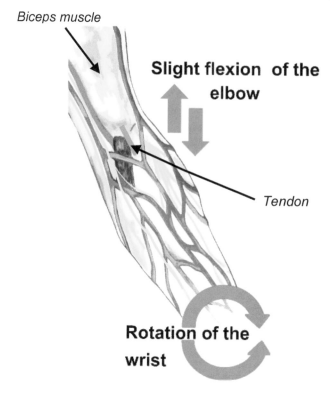

Slight flexion of the elbow

Tendon

Rotation of the wrist

Figure 58. Slightly flexing the elbow and or rotating the forearm can often help in locating suitable veins. With gentle flexion, the large central tendon from the biceps muscle can be felt.

The elbow should be slightly flexed. If the arm is held out straight, this can have the effect of pulling on the vein causing the lumen to narrow and flattening its appearance.

The forearm can also be rotated (palm uppermost or palm facing downwards). This sometimes has the effect of using the muscles in the arm to lift a vein upwards, pushing it into view.

The function of the tourniquet is to slow the flow of venous blood to facilitate venepuncture. It should not be so tight that it occludes the arterial flow and obliterates the pulse. If the tourniquet is applied too tightly, when the needle pierces the vein, the increased venous pressure can cause blood to spurt under the skin causing bruising.

Patients who have very thin skin may be more prone to bruising as there is very little tissue surrounding and supporting the vein. Where the patient has good veins but thin, papery skin, the tourniquet can be released immediately before venepuncture to lower the venous pressure.

To illustrate this point, consider a balloon. If it is over inflated the moment a pin is inserted the balloon goes 'bang' and splits. If it is inflated sufficiently to maintain its shape, a pin can be inserted and withdrawn and the air simply escapes. Thin-walled veins are very similar.

To locate more difficult veins, use the index finger of the non-dominant hand to intermittently press up and down on the vein. It should feel 'soft and bouncy'. Avoid asking the patient to open and close their fist or repeatedly tapping or slapping the potential site. Where access is particularly difficult, apply warm pads and hang the arm downwards to allow gravity to assist in filling the veins.

Applying the Tourniquet

Plain strip tourniquets are the least expensive and quick to tie once the technique has been mastered.

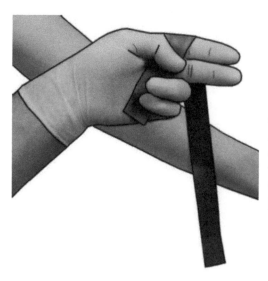

Figure 59. Hold two fingers out as illustrated and drape the tourniquet over the palm of the hand forming short and long limbs. The fingers should protrude as shown.

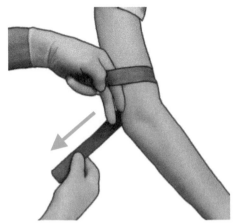

Figure 60. Drape the long limb over the arm and use the two straight fingers to push against the patients arm to prevent pinching the skin. Stretch the tourniquet in a downward direction.

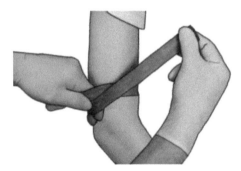

Figure 61. Bring the long limb upwards to cross over the short limb. Clamp the two limbs together using your thumb and index finger.

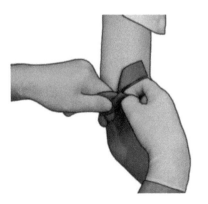

Figure 62. Grasping the two tourniquet limbs together, bend your fingers to create a space between the skin and tourniquet. Using the index finger as shown, tuck the tourniquet behind the band.

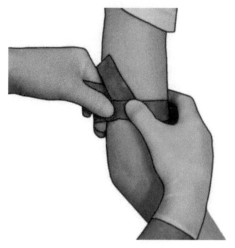

Figure 63. Hold the tourniquet in position with your thumb whilst you remove your fingers from behind the short limb.

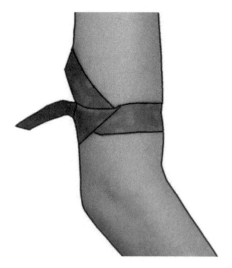

Figure 64. The tourniquet should lay flat on the arm with the tips of the short and long limbs protruding like ears from the top. The tourniquet is quickly released by gently tugging on the long limb on the right hand side.

The 'knot' should always be at the side of the arm. This prevents the protruding tourniquet tabs from falling onto the proposed puncture site risking contamination. This is also wise for male staff undertaking phlebotomy on female patients as attempts to remove a tourniquet located near the axilla could be misconstrued as inappropriate touching.

Hand hygiene should have been carried out and gloves put on in line with your Trust or institutional guidelines.

Many healthcare staff experience difficulties in palpating veins whilst wearing gloves. It is quite permissible to initially locate a vein with freshly gelled hands prior to prepping.

Prep the skin for 30 seconds and allow to air dry for a further 30 seconds. Do not re-palpate the proposed puncture site as this will re-contaminate the site. Where difficulty is encountered in locating the vein and re-palpation is considered essential, palpate above the proposed puncture site - never where the needle will enter the skin.

Apply the tourniquet. Keeping it flat on the skin prevents the band from rolling on removal thereby trapping and pulling on skin hairs which can be unpleasant for the patient.

TIP: Successful venepuncture often relies on being able to see a vein in your 'mind's eye'. When identifying a suitable vein, look for two marks on the skin over the vein which can be used as 'landmarks'. These may be freckles, little white, pink or brown blotches. By lining up the coloured hub of the needle with these two marks to produce a straight line over the vein, means one simply has to advance the needle in a downward direction. This technique reduces the incidence of missing those difficult veins.

Technique

There are no practical tests available to the phlebotomist to identify where the nerve runs. All that can be done is to choose wisely, avoid areas where nerves are known to be - such as alongside the basilic vein. Insert the needle at an angle of 15 – 25 degrees and never go deeper than is necessary, nor sweep the needle around under the skin in search of the vein. If you have missed withdraw the needle slightly so that the tip is just under the skin, redirect it and advance into the vein.

Larger patients who are well covered in adipose tissue are more difficult as the veins are located more deeply. Naturally, the needle needs to penetrate a little further.

When removing the needle sheath, do so with one straight movement. Attempts at loosening the sheath before removal can cause a small barb to form at the needle tip causing pain when the needle is removed.

Holding the arm gently but firmly, apply gentle traction on the surrounding tissue with the thumb. This ensures the skin is taught and the needle passes through the skin easily, quickly bypassing the pain nerve endings. Traction on the skin with the thumb can also help to straighten curved or tortuous veins.

At the moment of venepuncture, slight pressure with the thumb can take the patient's mind off the needle puncture: they are expecting a 'sharp scratch' but not pressure. Done correctly, it is difficult for the patient to determine whether the pressure or the scratch is the most prominent of sensations.

When performing venepuncture, have an imaginary line which only the needle crosses. Logically, if you are always behind the needle, you cannot get a needlestick. Additionally, this gives a clear field of view of the puncture site and surrounding area.

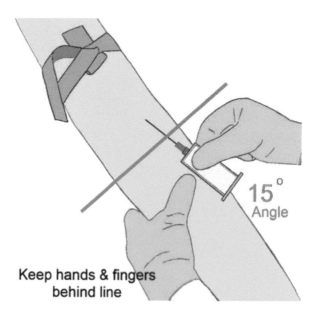

Figure 65. The imaginary line which the phlebotomist should always aim to be behind. This provides a clear view of the procedure site.

Note how the needle holder is held in the diagram. This provides clear visual access to the puncture site and allows the needle to enter the skin at the correct angle of 15 to 25 degrees.

Phlebotomy needles are ground to have a cutting edge which helps to minimise pain on entry and for this reason never sweep around under the skin searching for a vein or rotate the needle within a vein.

Generally, it is advised to use the same hand to support the needle holder as was used to insert it. However, where the room and equipment layout requires the phlebotomist to cross over arms to reach equipment, the holder should be transferred into the non- dominant hand thus allowing the phlebotomist to easily pick up tubes and swabs without crossing hands. This is particularly important when it comes to disposing of used sharps when there can be a real risk of injury.

Rest the index and middle finger on the patients arm and place a thumb on top of the holder. If the patient moves slightly, the practitioner moves with the patient's arm more easily thereby ensuring the needle does not slip out of the vein. Never hold the device in position by placing a finger or thumb over the needle at the puncture site.

Attaching and Changing Tubes
Following the Order of Draw, attach the tubes with the label downwards. This allows you to see directly into the tube to ensure it is filling and determine the volume collected. Tubes should always fill from the bottom upwards.

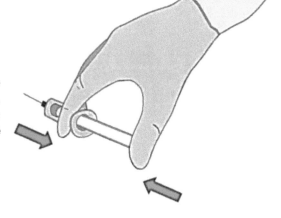

Figure 66. Using the flanges on the holder, squeeze the tube onto the multi-sample needle.

By squeezing the tube on, as shown (Figure 66.) the force of pushing the tube is counteracted by pulling back against the needle holder flange thus maintaining the needle's position in the vein.

Once blood starts flowing into the tube, the tourniquet should be released to ensure a free-flowing sample is obtained. Remember the maximum time for the tourniquet is one minute.

When changing tubes, the pull on the tube is counteracted by pushing against the needle holder. These opposite forces balance each other out and prevent the needle coming out of the vein.

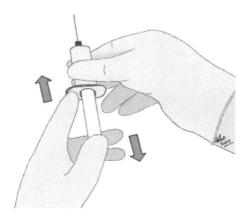

Figure 67. Technique for withdrawing sample tubes. Opposite forces counteract each other maintaining the needle's position in the vein.

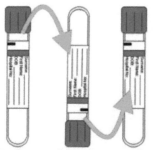

As each tube is withdrawn, slowly and gently invert it several times to ensure the sample is well mixed with any tube additive. It must not be shaken or exposed to vigorous exertion as there is the risk of damaging the blood cells.

1 Complete Inversion

Figure 68. Slowly and gently invert the sample tube to ensure the blood is well mixed with any tube additive.

After the last tube is filled, remove it from the holder and cover the puncture site with a cotton swab but do not press at this stage otherwise the needle cuts the skin and possibly the vein on withdrawal causing pain or discomfort to the patient. Apply pressure when the needle is clear of the skin.

Operate the needle guard as recommended by the device manufacturer – usually either with the thumb or a convenient flat surface. Dispose of the sharp immediately in the sharps container.

Winged Collection Sets

These devices can be used at any normal phlebotomy site but due to their cost they are generally reserved for more difficult venepunctures and when using the dorsal veins of the hand.

Ordinary multi-sample needles should never be used when collecting blood from the back of the hand due to the gauge of the needle and especially the length. It is easy with a long needle to damage tendons in the hand.

Winged sets have an advantage that once they have entered the vein, a small amount of blood flows into the tubing (flashback) confirming correct placement. Once inserted, there is no need for them to be taped in place: a thumb from the same or opposite hand can hold one wing against the skin while the holder is tucked into the palm of the same hand. This gives the phlebotomist one free hand to attach and remove sample tubes, release the tourniquet and apply a swab to the puncture site while the other hand carries out all functions of the collection set including operating the safety guard.

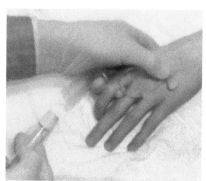

Figure 69. Holding a winged collection set and holder giving a free hand to handle tubes, release the tourniquet and apply a swab.

As the needles on winged sets tend to be much shorter than conventional multi-sample needles, they should be inserted a little further into the vein if possible as they can dislodge easily.

When inserting a winged set, the non-dominant hand of the phlebotomist performs several functions apart from simply holding the patients hand still: the thumb is used to stretch the skin to stabilise the vein and the finger-tips can be placed into the palm of the patients hand and slight upward pressure can raise the vein up so that the back of the hand is relatively flat. This helps prevent the needle from wandering.

Good tension on the skin helps the needle penetrate more quickly thereby reducing the discomfort.

When inserting the needle into tortuous veins which cannot be straightened by skin tension alone, the winged set can be repeatedly shuffled from left to right to advance it further into the vein.

The underside of the wings have a roughened surface so the winged set can be grasped securely when wearing gloves. When inserting these devices, always ensure you are able to clearly see the flashback chamber.

Discard Tube

When taking coagulation or other volume sensitive samples, air in the winged set tubing will enter the sample tube causing it to slightly under fill. This can be overcome by attaching either a plain or identical citrate tube first to drawn off the air. Once there is a splash of blood in the tube it should be removed, discarded into the sharps container and the sample tube attached.

Problem solving

Occasionally, like any other clinical procedure, things do not go as planned. What seems to be a simple procedure at the start can easily turn up difficulties which, once the reasons are understood, become easier to resolve.

Blood Fails to Flow

There are several reasons why blood fails to flow into the tube. The first is of course that the needle has failed to penetrate the vein.

Consider whether this may be the case and if so, partially withdrawn the needle, redirect it and advance the needle into the vein.

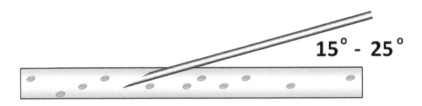

Figure 70. A normal venepuncture. The vein is large enough to allow blood to flow.

Occasionally, the bevel of the needle may sit under the cusp of a valve within the vein and applying the vacuum tube draws the valve down over the bevel preventing entry of blood.

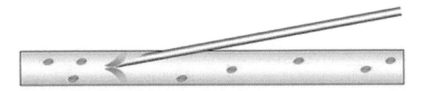

Figure 71. Showing the bezel of the needle against a valve which impedes blood flow into the tube.

Where this happens, remove the sample tube and attempt to reposition the needle. Occasionally, the needle can be gently advanced or pulled back to clear the valve. Re-apply the sample tube but consider re-siting the needle if blood still fails to flow.

Collapsed Veins

Occasionally veins are said to 'collapse' and blood flow ceases. This is usually caused by operator error in using too large a needle in too small a vein so that blood is prevented from passing the needle and entering the bevelled needle opening.

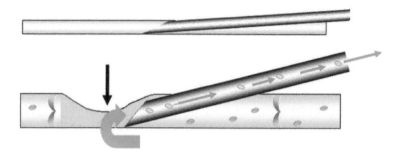

Figure 72. A 'Collapsed' vein. A needle which is too large for a small vein prevents blood passing the needle before it can be drawn into the lumen. The tube vacuum pulls the vein wall over the bevel thus occluding the lumen.

Occasionally, a collapsed vein can be remedied by very gently lifting the whole needle vertically by a millimetre or so. Take care not to lever as the needle tip can easily puncture the vein.

Transfixion
This is where the needle passes through the vein and protrudes through the back wall. This is easily identified when a tube is attached as a small amount of blood - collected as the needle passed through the vein - is sprayed into the tube. This can easily occur when the angle of insertion is above 25 degrees from the horizontal plane. Simply withdrawing the needle slightly soon remedies this problem.

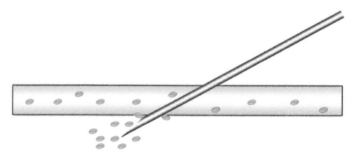

Figure 73. Vein transfixed by needle as it protrudes through the posterior wall.

Rolling Veins

Veins which lack good supportive tissue can easily move and roll making insertion of the needle into the lumen difficult. This is more evident in thick walled veins that perhaps show some signs of calcification. Ensuring good traction on the skin helps stabilise the vein.

Drinking plenty of water & other myths

Often where phlebotomists have been unable to obtain a sample, patients are told to drink plenty of fluids before their next appointment in the belief that this will help to swell the veins and make the phlebotomist's task easier.

In one incident, the phlebotomist having failed to obtain a sample advised a patient to drink two litres of water before returning the following day. This is a considerable amount of water to drink in one go. It will add to the patient's distress and will not help fill the veins in the slightest - unless the patient is grossly dehydrated by 2 Litres or more. Even then, rehydration requires a more gradual approach and is best performed in the light of blood results (which at this stage have yet to be obtained) and under the direction of a medical practitioner.

The reason why this fails to work is that the patient has kidneys and a bladder which are working constantly to regulate fluid balance. All that happens is the poor patient has a dire need to repeatedly void urine and the inability to do so while travelling to the hospital or clinic, only adds further anxiety causing peripheral veins to shut down.

If drinking a large volume of water instantly made its way into the circulatory system, the blood results would be hugely abnormal in any event because the average blood volume of 5 Litres would have been diluted by an additional 40% volume.

The best advice to the patient is to wear warm clothing and keep their arms well covered. This causes venous dilation revealing veins which are more easily accessed.

How to be a good phlebotomist

The trick to being a good phlebotomist is to pay attention to detail, look for errors not just confirmation. Check and check again.

When first starting out, take your time with patients and don't be rushed into attempting the venepuncture until you are sure you have located a good vein and in a position where trauma and nerve injury are unlikely. There is nothing worse than failure to deflate confidence.

Most hospitals have a policy which states that if you miss it is permissible to have another one or two attempts. Before you have a second attempt, ask yourself whether you are likely to succeed. If you have missed on your first choice of vein, will you be more successful on your second choice? If the answer is no, forgo another attempt and pass this draw onto a more experienced colleague.

When presented with difficult draws, there is no shame is passing it on to someone more experienced – one day your juniors will do the same and pass their difficult draws over to you and it is important to work within your level of competency.

Most patients will respect your honesty and judgement in seeking assistance. Indeed many patients know from previous visits to the phlebotomy clinic that they are difficult. If you fail today, the next time the patient presents themselves for their blood test, they remember that you couldn't get it last time (so do you) and your confidence takes another battering. Of course sometimes you will miss – everybody does sometimes. It is just that as you gain experience, you learn to recognise and avoid those veins that you know you will not get and find another that you know you will.

Whenever the opportunity presents, observe an experienced colleague tackle those trickier veins. Ask them to explain their choices and why and what they do to ensure success. With regular practice you will gain experience and you will improve rapidly.

With this new found level of skill, a quiet, confident and professional approach to patients' should follow. Showing compassion and appreciation of their fears and anxiety will put you in good stead with most patients you are likely to encounter.

Difficult Patients – Faints & Phobias

Many individuals have a fear of needles or of seeing blood and may exhibit a wide range of emotions. Remain calm and professional. If possible discuss their fears and together plan an approach that will permit the sample to be obtained. Some patients do not object to the blood test – it is the needle they cannot bear to see. If so, plan a way that prevents this. Others may fear pain they associate with needles. In these instances, a topical local anaesthetic cream such as EMLA™ or Ametop™ can be prescribed and applied to the proposed puncture site and covered with a clear waterproof dressing for about an hour to ensure the skin is numb.

Remember a phobia may be an irrational fear but they are very real and distressing to the patient. It is important to build a good rapport and trust and to agree on a solution or at least a compromise which enables the sample to be taken. The patient must remain in complete control and be sure that nothing will happen until they are ready and if they say 'Stop', the request will be obeyed.

Where patients have a history of fainting always arrange for them to lie down while the sample is taken.

Fainting is caused by a sudden fall in blood pressure caused by the *Vagus nerve* acting like a brake on the heart rate. Because the heart beat slows, it is unable to circulate blood to the brain and so the patient passes out. This is often called a *vaso-vagal* attack.

Nature's own remedy is that by collapsing, the heart only has to circulate blood horizontally, thereby restoring circulation to the brain. The blood pressure returns to normal and the patient recovers. It is important not to let the patient stand for several minutes.

When a patient faints, call for help and abandon the procedure. Tilt the phlebotomy chair into a slightly head down position to help raise their blood pressure. If the chair does not tilt, try to lower their head. This can be difficult in obese patients as they often do not bend that far and in this position, breathing can become more difficult. Ensure the patient cannot fall or sustain any injury.

Where there is no other alternative, the patient may need to be laid on the floor to recover. If they are large, assistance will be required. Ensure a pillow is placed under the head.

In some instances – especially with patients with learning difficulties or phobias, it may be advantageous for the patient to visit the phlebotomy department informally, sit in the chair and have a tourniquet lightly applied and their skin prepped. No sample is taken at this stage, it is just a casual visit which allows them to experience the routine, meet their phlebotomist in safety thereby building their confidence.

Transporting Specimens

Blood specimens should always be transported to the laboratory in leak-proof containers and consideration given to environmental factors such as extremes of temperature or bright sunlight. Cold can raise potassium by causing it to leach from the cells while excessive heat can de-nature proteins – in effect slow cook the sample whilst direct sunlight breaks down bilirubin. Samples for ammonia should be transported on ice while samples for cryoglobulins should be kept at body temperature of $37°$ Centigrade. A metal thermos flask is ideal for these purposes in that it can hold iced water or be preheated to body temperature.

Transportation may be by the phlebotomist, a porter, via a pneumatic air tube system or in some instances by post to specialist laboratories.

Samples such as those for the Clozapine Patient Monitoring Service (Clozaril™) are sent via Royal Mail. The sample must be packaged in Post Office approved packaging. The sample having been correctly labelled is wrapped in a lint material to absorb the blood should a leak occur. This is then placed into a clam-shell plastic box and placed in a sealable plastic bag which together with the form, is placed into a pre-addressed plastic self-seal envelope.

Samples transported by car should be in a leak-proof container clearly marked 'Bio-Hazard'.

Advice to the Patient after a blood test

After obtaining a blood sample, advise the patient not to bend their elbow as this raises the pressure in the vein and causes bruising. They should also refrain from lifting or carrying heavy items for at least half an hour and remember to remove the plaster or dressing.

The Sample Journey

The following table outlines the basic steps and stages in the sample journey from generation of the Request Form to dispatching the sample to the laboratory.

Table 6. THE PHLEBOTOMY SAMPLE JOURNEY

Request Form	Generated by Doctor or other Healthcare Professional	Hand Written / Computer Printed	Verified
Patient Identification Checked by Phlebotomist	Open Questions Verbal	ID Band Verified	Matched against Form
Sample Obtained	Skin Prep 30 seconds prep / 30 seconds dry	Tourniquet 1 minute maximum	Single use Gloves
Label Tube(s)	Details from ID Band (In-Patient) or Request form (Out-Patient)	Matched to Request Form	Matched to patient
Re-Check tube & form	4 PID	Date / Time	Sign
Send to Laboratory	Within appropriate time	Appropriately packaged	Avoid Extremes of Temperature. Sunlight/ Cold or Heat

Summary of Phlebotomy Procedure

1. Introduce yourself to the patient and gain valid consent.
2. Identify the patient correctly using appropriate points of ID.
3. Perform Hand Hygiene.
4. Select a suitable vein.
5. Ensure Intravenous infusions are not running into the same arm.
6. Prep the skin as per your Trust policy.
7. Apply a tourniquet 10 cm above the proposed puncture site.
8. Wear well-fitting gloves.
9. Apply traction to the skin to stabilise the vein.
10. Insert the needle gently into the vein at an angle of 15 – 25 degrees depending on how close the vein lies to the surface.
11. Following the Order of Draw, insert the first tube with the label downwards. Squeeze the tube on as shown in Figure 66.
12. When blood flows into the tube, release the tourniquet.
13. Remove sample tube as shown in Figure 67.
14. Invert sample tubes 5 or 6 times (or as recommended) to ensure the specimen is well mixed with any tube additive such as EDTA or citrate.
15. Gently cover the puncture site with a swab and withdraw the needle.
16. Apply pressure to the puncture site. The patient may do this if they are willing and able to do so but must be monitored by the phlebotomist.
17. Dispose of sharps and other clinical waste.
18. Apply a suitable dressing.
19. Label the sample from the ID Band (In-Patient) or Request Form (Out-Patient).
20. Remove gloves and discard in clinical waste container.
21. Perform hand hygiene.
22. Thank the patient and assist them as necessary.

Never USE Pre-Labelled Tubes

BLOOD CULTURES 12

Blood cultures are acknowledged as the 'gold standard' in the diagnosis of blood borne infections as they enable the causative organism to be identified and the most appropriate and effective antibiotic to be prescribed. The results are particularly important to the Microbiology and Infection Control Departments as there is a requirement to report some results such as MRSA and *Clostridium difficile* to the Department of Health.

It is essential that these reports are not distorted by the inclusion of poorly obtained and contaminated samples as it suggests that the hospital's infection control is lacking. It is therefore important that blood culture samples are taken using a strictly aseptic technique.

Blood culture bottles are usually packed as pairs: one for the culture and growth of aerobic bacteria such as MRSA and the other for culturing anaerobic bacteria such as *Clostridium difficile*.

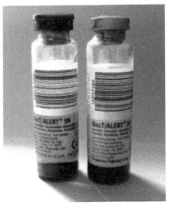

Aerobic bacteria are those which can only replicate in the presence of oxygen. Anaerobic bacteria are those which only replicate in the absence of oxygen.

Allowing air to contaminate the anaerobic sample can cause really fastidious bacteria to form spores which is their dormant, inactive state. Dormancy prevents the bacteria from respiring and therefore cannot be detected by normal laboratory blood culture procedure.

Figure 74. A pair of BacT/ALERT Blood Culture Bottles - bioMérieux.

Culture bottles contain sterile tryptic soy protein - a nutrient broth which provides bacteria in the sample sufficient nutrients to enable them to survive and multiply.

In the base of the bottles is a coloured indicator disc which should be a greenish blue colour. If bacteria are present and replicating, they produce carbon dioxide which interacts with the chemical indicator disc changing the colour to yellow.

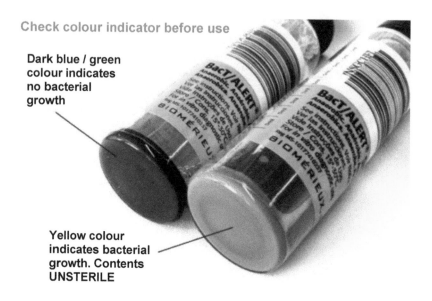

Check colour indicator before use

Dark blue / green colour indicates no bacterial growth

Yellow colour indicates bacterial growth. Contents UNSTERILE

Figure 75. Check the colorimetric indictor disc in the base of the sample bottles. Discard any bottles where the disc is yellow or discoloured.

Culture bottles should have coloured plastic tops which form a seal covering the puncture membrane. These seals do not guarantee the sterility of the rubber membrane; rather they are **Tamper Evident Seals.** Their purpose is simply to show that the bottles have not previously been inoculated. The coloured indicator disc in the base indicates that the contents remain sterile.

Before use, always check the colour of the indicator disc, expiry date and tamper evident seals discarding any which are discoloured, out-of-date or, where the seals are missing.

The volume of blood collected for culture is a very significant factor in detecting organisms and a direct relationship exists between the blood volume collected and bacterial yield. Ideally in adults, each bottle should be filled with at least 10 mls of blood. This may seem rather severe but the bacterial count in the bloodstream may only amount to 1 bacterium per 3 mls of blood. It follows therefore that there may only be 3 or 4 bacteria in total in the sample bottle. Under filled bottles can easily result in no bacteria present producing false negative results (Connell *et al*).

To measure the volume of blood entering the bottles, a scale is printed on the edge of the label.

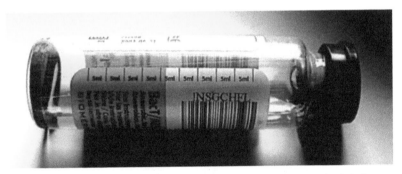

Figure 76. A blood culture bottle showing the filling scale on the label.

When obtaining blood culture samples, the bottles must be held in the upright position. The rationale behind this is that the medium is a chemical additive - not a prescription medicine and therefore it must never come into direct contact with an indwelling needle. Additionally, the medium may carry over into the next sample tube causing erroneous results.

These points of carefully checking the indicator discs, tamper evident seals and ensuring the bottles are held upright when sampling cannot be over stressed as a contaminated bottle producing a healthy colony of bacteria will also be producing a good amount of carbon dioxide. This will cause the bottle to become pressurised and if attached to a needle in a patient, this pressure would inject the contaminated medium intravenously with disastrous results.

The patient may suffer as a result of the medium but may also suffer from toxic shock as a result of the huge number of bacteria injected as a bolus. It is these points which dictate that blood cultures deserve a separate chapter and are only obtained by staff who have received appropriate training and competency assessment.

Many hospitals now have a strict policy regarding blood culture collection and in most cases, it is recommended that two sets of cultures are obtained at least 20 minutes apart and from different sites. This not only increases the yield of causative bacteria but can also determine whether the previous sample was contaminated.

Some hospitals utilise sterile blood culture packs, others may simply use sterile pre-packed items which are readily available in their ward treatment rooms.

The following illustrations (Figures 77 – 88) are intended as a guide to the principles of collecting blood cultures but practitioners must always follow their own Trust policy and guidelines.

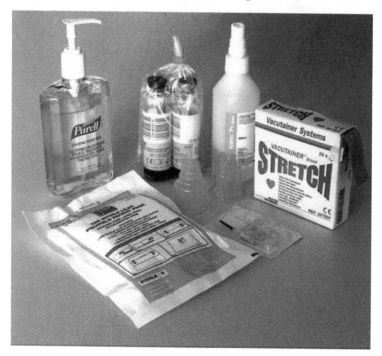

Figure 77. Gather all equipment to prevent interruptions to the procedure.

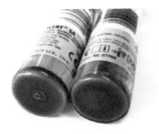

Figure 78. Check colorimetric indictor disc to ensure sterility.

Check expiry date. Check tamper evident seals are intact. Discard any bottles which do not conform.

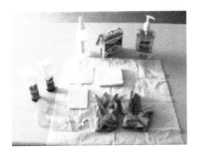

Figure 79. Open sterile pack and tip winged collection set onto sterile field.

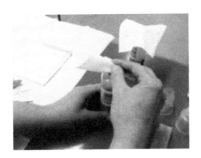

Figure 80. Remove tamper evident seals and prepare culture bottles by cleaning tops. Leave covered with a sterile swab until ready to use. Use a fresh swab for each bottle.

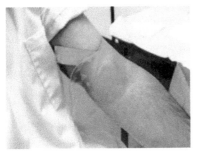

Figure 81. Apply tourniquet and select suitable vein.

Thoroughly clean the skin in a spiral motion with 2% Chlorhexidine and 70% Isopropyl alcohol for at least 30 seconds and allow a further 30 seconds to air dry. Never try to speed up the drying process by swabbing, fanning or blowing on the site. Proprietary brands such as Chloraprep™ or Hydrex™ solution are often used.

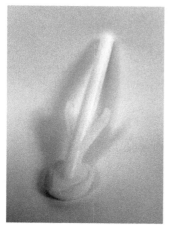

Figure 82. Chloraprep™ suitable for cleansing the proposed puncture site. The two side arms when squeezed together break open an ampoule of 2% Chlorhexidine and 70% isopropyl alcohol which soaks the sponge ready for use.

Other more simpler Chloroprep™ devices are also available.

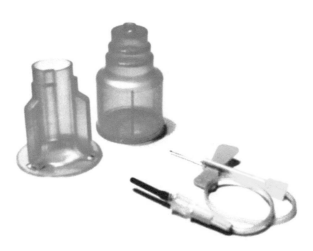

Figure 83. Prepare or assemble winged collection set with large culture bottle needle holder. A safety guard insert (left) is available where other routine samples are to be obtained.

Pre-assembled collection sets are much more convenient as both the holder and winged set are sterile and can be handled without fear of de-sterilising the practitioner's gloves. However, where the sterile winged collection set must be assembled with a non-sterile holder, a simple method is to put on one sterile glove with which to hold the winged set and grasp the unsterile holder with the un-gloved hand. Once these are assembled the device can be placed on the edge of the sterile field and the other glove can then be put on. Only handle the device by the sterile wings.

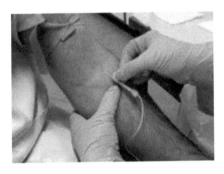

Figure 84. Perform vene-puncture using a strictly aseptic technique.

A sterile paper towel can be placed over the arm to maintain sterility of the practitioner's gloves.

Once the winged set has been placed in the vein using a strict aseptic technique, the practitioner can then handle the unsterile bottle exteriors and tourniquet. However, when handling the bottles, be sure never to touch the 'prepped' inoculating membrane.

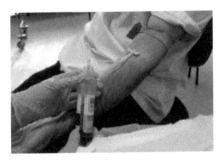

Figure 85. Hold culture bottles upright, obtaining **AEROBIC** sample first followed by the **ANAEROBIC** bottle.

When taking cultures the luer adaptor should not be disconnected from the tubing to allow blood flow to eliminate air in the line: the air trapped in the tubing is sterile and will not contaminate the aerobic sample nor prevent bacterial growth. Exposing the line to room air just may allow the ingress of extraneous bacteria which could cause contamination if they are able to replicate.

Use the filling gauge located on the bottle label to measure the blood volume obtained. The gap in the label also allows good visibility of blood flow.

Once the aerobic sample has been obtained, blood flow will have eliminated the air in the line. The anaerobic bottle can now be attached without fear of introducing air which may inhibit bacterial growth.

The tourniquet should now be removed and if other samples are required for biochemistry or haematology, the aperture reducing guard should be inserted. This prevents the practitioner's fingers from potential injury in the event they inadvertently slip into the holder onto the multi-sample luer adaptor needle.

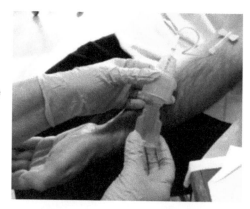

Figure 86. Inserting the aperture reducing guard.

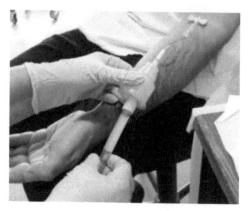

Figure 87. With the guard in place, other samples may now taken.

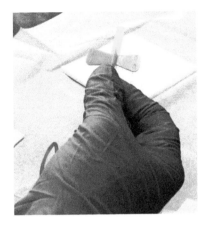

Figure 88. The safety guard is operated with one hand by gripping the tubing with the fingers and pushing the guard held between thumb and index finger. The winged set and holder are now ready to place into the sharps container.

Label all tubes at the patient's bedside taking the details from the Identity Band or using a bar-code scanner from the ID Band.

Transport the samples to the laboratory maintaining room temperature immediately after collection and in any event within 4 hours (Public Health England). Blood cultures should never be placed in a refrigerator as the cold temperature will inhibit bacterial growth and may even destroy the few bacteria that have been obtained.

The only samples which are routinely placed in a refrigerator are urine samples. The cold temperature will inhibit bacterial growth but it also inhibits contaminant bacteria from overgrowth which could lead them to appear to be the causative organism.

Blood Cultures – Syringe & Needle Technique

Although using a syringe and needle to obtain samples is far from ideal in terms of health and safety – i.e. piercing a rubber stopper with the hollow bore needle used to obtain the sample, attached to a syringe full of potentially infected blood is an outdated and dangerous practice and one which no healthcare worker should be required to do - yet a number of institutions still use this technique.

If a syringe and needle must be used, the order of filling the bottles is reversed – anaerobic should be filled first followed by aerobic. This ensures any air in the form of bubbles in the syringe do not find their way into the anaerobic bottle.

References & Further Reading

1. Stefani S. Diagnostic techniques in bloodstream infections: where are we going? Int J Antimicrob Agents 2009; 34 Suppl 4:S9-12.

2. Kelly MT, Roberts FJ, Henry D, Geere I, Smith JA. Clinical comparison of isolator and BACTEC 660 resin media for blood culture. J Clin Microbiol 1990; 28:1925-7.

3. Connell TG, Rele M, Cowley D, Buttery JP, Curtis N. How reliable is a negative blood culture result? Volume of blood submitted for culture in routine practice in a children's hospital. Pediatrics 2007; 119:891-6.

4. Mermel LA, Maki DG. Detection of bacteremia in adults: consequences of culturing an inadequate volume of blood. Ann Intern Med 1993; 119:270-2.

5. Public Health England. (2014). Investigation of Blood Cultures (for Organisms other than *Mycobacterium* species). UK Standards for Microbiology Investigations. B 37 Issue 8. Available from - https://www.gov.uk/uk-standards-for-microbiology- investigations-smi-quality-and-consistency-in-clinical- laboratories.

Common Blood Tests and their Abbreviations

APTR   Activated partial thromboplastin ratio –
             a blood clotting test. Often used when
             patients are receiving heparin.

APTT   Activated partial thromboplastin time
             – a test of blood clotting. Often used
             when patients are receiving heparin.

Cross Match   Blood sample for matching to Group
             specific (ABO & Rhesus) blood. Often 2
             samples are required for routine
             transfusions.

Differential Count   Some infections cause an increase in
             certain types of White Blood Cells which
             may give clues to the specific cause such
             as whether an infection is caused by
             bacteria, virus or fungi.

ESR   **Erythrocyte Sedimentation Rate** –
             is based on the rate at which red blood
             cells (erythrocytes) fall and settle in a
             test tube. In infections, if antibodies
             have bound to the red cells they are
             larger, heavier and settle much faster.

FBC   **Full Blood Count** - this is a series of
             tests, assessing red cell numbers to
             check for anaemia, white cell count to
             check for infection, platelets for clotting
             disorders and red cell indices such as
             haemoglobin, and cell size.

Group & Screen **Group & Screen** - The ABO and Rhesus groups are identified and the sample stored temporarily.

I.N.R **International Normalised Ratio** – a coagulation test for patients on the warfarin type anticoagulants. Using an internationally standardised test permits holiday makers to have their warfarin level checked and prescribed whilst abroad.

Kleihaeur Used to measure the amount of foetal haemoglobin transferred to the mother's bloodstream - usually for Rhesus-negative mothers to determine the dose of anti-D.

Monospot / Infectious Mononucleosis/ Paul Bunnel A specific test for infectious mononucleosis or glandular fever caused by the Epstein-Barr Virus.

Biochemistry

Albumin A large plasma protein which acts as a carrier for other substances in the blood. Usually altered in liver or renal disease or may be low in digestive disorders.

Bilirubin Bilirubin is the yellowish-brown pigment released as red blood cells are broken down. Usually increased in cases of haemolysis or where the bile duct is obstructed for example by gall-stones.

Cholesterol A waxy substance – 80% produced in the liver the remainder is ingested in foods. Cholesterol is essential for good health and is a precursor to some hormones such as testosterone. High Density = the good cholesterol – Low Density termed the bad cholesterol. Fasting is unnecessary prior to blood testing.

Creatinine A waste product of metabolism especially muscle.

Creatine (CK) Also known as creatine phosphokinase (CPK). CK is an enzyme present in many tissues especially cardiac muscle, skeletal muscle and the brain.

C-RP **C-Reactive Protein** – an acute phase reactant produced in the liver. The C-RP closely follows infections – rapidly rising and falling.

D-dimer A test often performed for deep vein thrombosis, pulmonary embolism and myocardial infarction. The D-dimer is a degradation product of blood coagulation.

Glucose Fasting Glucose is used as the diagnostic test for diabetes. Random glucose tests are used for monitoring.

GGT / γGT **Gamma-glutamyl transferase** – or **Gamma GT** – an enzyme found in many tissues, especially the liver. Used as an indicator of hepatitis or excessive alcohol consumption.

Protein Protein is derived from the digestive system and can be low in instances of malnutrition or renal disease.

PSA **Prostate Specific Antigen** – a marker for prostatic carcinoma. To avoid falsely elevated results, the blood sample should be taken prior to physical examination of the prostate gland.

TFTs **Thyroid Function** – Thyroid Simulating Hormone is produced by the pituitary gland and controls activity. T3 & T4 are produced by the thyroid gland and under production can result in hypothyroidism

(Myxoedema) whilst over production can result in hyperthyroidism (thyrotoxicosis).

U & Es   **Urea & Electrolytes** – a routine biochemistry test for Urea and electrolytes such as sodium and potassium. The test shows results for hydration and renal function.

Glossary of Terms

Anterior The front surface when viewing the body from the front with palms facing forwards. The front face of an organ or tissue.

Bacteraemia The presence of bacteria in the blood stream causing a severe infection. *Also called Septicaemia.*

Cannula A small gauge plastic tube inserted into a vein for the purpose of infusing sterile solutions such as saline, transfusing blood or blood products or injecting intravenous medication.

Clot Activator A substance such as silica which is added to phlebotomy tubes to promote blood clotting.

COSHH Control Of Substances Hazardous to Health. COSHH is the law which regulates and governs the use, storage and handling of hazardous substances.

CVC Central Venous Catheter. A catheter inserted usually in a neck vein into the central veins in the chest.

Cytotoxic Material, especially drugs which are toxic to tissue cells. Waste from these items must be destroyed by incineration.

Dwarfism Genetic abnormality resulting in short stature.

Fomite An inanimate object which can carry infective material.

Giantism	Excessive growth in stature o f t e n caused by over secretion of growth hormone from the pituitary gland.
Haematoma	A collection of blood under the skin which causes a swelling. This may take several weeks to subside.
Haemoconcentration	An increase in cellular and other blood components due to prolonged tourniquet time.
Haemolysis	*(Haem* = Blood + *lysis* = breakdown). The breakdown or rupturing of red blood cells. This releases potassium and the pigment *haem* into the plasma. Thus haemolysed samples are unsuitable for haematology or biochemistry testing.
Hepatitis	Inflammation of the liver – usually due to viral infection by Hepatitis. A, B, C, D, or E.
Hypertension	High blood pressure. (Hypertensive).
Hyperkalaemia	A high blood potassium level which can affect the contractility of the heart.
Hypokalaemia the heart.	A low blood potassium level. This condition can affect the contractility of
Hypotension	Low blood pressure.
Mastectomy	Removal of a breast. Although usually females, males can also develop breast cancer and require a mastectomy.
Mucocutaneous	Absorbed through a mucous membrane. Mucocutaneous exposure – risk of infection by a blood borne virus

Mucous membrane	The lining to the mouth and gut, respiratory and urinary tracts.
Nosocomial	An infection taking place or originating in a hospital or healthcare environment.
Oedema	Retention of fluid in the tissues causing affected tissue to become swollen. Common in the feet and ankles where it is known as peripheral oedema. Can also occur in lungs - pulmonary oedema or brain – cerebral oedema.
Pathogens	Bacterial, viral, fungal and parasitic organisms which are capable of causing disease.
PEP	Post Exposure Prophylaxis – the medication used to treat HIV is given to those who have had a needlestick injury where there is a risk of contact with HIV.
Percutaneous	Through the skin. Percutaneous injury – where the skin has been puncture by a needle or broken by other sharp objects. Scratches and bites are included in the definition.
Phlebitis	Inflammation of a vein. This may be through bacterial infection or reaction to chemicals and medication.
Phlebotomy	The term used to denote obtaining a blood specimen intravenously for the express purpose of analysis.

PICC Line — Peripherally Inserted Central Catheter. A long thin flexible tube inserted into a peripheral vein such as in the arm with its distal end in the superior vena cava.

Posterior — The body viewed from the back with the palms facing forwards. The back of an organ or tissue.

RIDDOR — Reporting of Injuries, Diseases and Dangerous Occurrences Regulations 2013.

Septicaemia — A severe infection where bacteria in the blood are circulated to all tissues and organs.

Thixotropic — The term used to describe the serum separator gel used in biochemistry tubes which forms a barrier between the cells and serum. The gel liquefies during centrifugation and being lighter than cells, rises up the tube and sits on top. It resets to a gel once it is left to stand.

Thrombophlebitis — Inflammation of a vein (phlebitis) in conjunction with the formation of a blood clot (Thrombus)

VAD — Venous Access Device. A general term to describe all intravenous access devices such as cannulae, mid-lines and long lines etc.

Venepuncture — The act of inserting a needle or cannula into a vein.

Venesection — Venepuncture with the purpose of removing a predetermined volume of blood to treat conditions such as iron overload.

Common Abbreviations

ABGs	Arterial Blood Gases
ABO	Blood Grouping classification
ADH	Anti diuretic Hormone
AHCS	Academy for Healthcare Science
Ag	Antigen
ALP	Alkaline phosphatase
ANA	Antinuclear antibody
APTR	Activated partial thromboplastin ratio
APTT	Activated partial thromboplastin time
AST	Aspartate Transaminase
BMS	Bio-Medical Scientist
BNP	Brain naturetic peptide
BP	Blood pressure
BUN	Blood Urea Nitrogen
Ca	Chemical symbol for Calcium
CABG	Coronary Artery Bypass Graft
CEA	Carcino-embryonic antigen
CK	Creatine kinase
CK-MB	Creatine kinase isoenzyme MB
CK-MM	Creatine kinase isoenzyme MM
Cl	Chemical symbol for chloride or chlorine
CMV	Cytomegalovirus
CNS	Central nervous system
CO	Chemical symbol for carbon monoxide
CO_2	Chemical symbol for carbon dioxide
COPD	Chronic Obstructive Pulmonary Disease
COSHH	Control of substances hazardous to health
CPA	Clinical Pathology Accreditation
CPMS	Clozaril Patient Monitoring Service
CPR	Cardiopulmonary resuscitation
CQC	Care Quality Commission
C-RP	C-Reactive Protein
C & S	Culture and Sensitivity
CSF	Cerebro-spinal fluid
CVA	Cerebrovascular accident
DIC	Disseminated intravascular coagulation
DM	Diabetes mellitus
EBV	Epstein-Barr Virus
ECG	Electro-Cardio Graph
EDTA	Ethylene-diamine-tetra-acetic acid
ESR	Erythrocyte Sedimentation Rate

ETOH	Shorthand abbreviation for ethyl-alcohol (Alcoholic drink)
FDP	Fibrin degradation product
Fe	Chemical symbol for iron
FSH	Follicle Stimulating Hormone
FUO	Fever of unknown origin
GGT	Gamma Glutamyl transferase
G & S	Group & Screen
GUM	Genito-Urinary Medicine
Hb	Haemoglobin
HBsAg	Hepatitis B virus surface antigen
Hep B	Hepatitis B virus
Hep C	Hepatitis C virus
HDL	High-density lipoprotein
HIV	Human Immunodeficiency Virus
HSE	Health & Safety Executive
HTA	Human Tissue Authority
INR	International Normalised Ratio
K	Chemical symbol for potassium
KOH	Potassium hydroxide
K_2-EDTA	Di-potassium ethylene-diamine-tetra-acetic acid
K_3-EDTA	Tri-potassium ethylene-diamine-tetra-acetic acid
Kg	Kilogram
LDH	Lactate Dehydrogenase
LDL	Low-density lipoprotein
LFTs	Liver function tests
LH	Luteinising hormone
Li	Chemical symbol for Lithium
MCH	Mean corpuscular haemoglobin
MCHC	Mean corpuscular haemoglobin concentration
MCV	Mean corpuscular volume
MHRA	Medicines & Healthcare Products Regulatory Agency
MI	Myocardial infarction
Mg	Chemical symbol for magnesium
mg	Milligram
MRI	Magnetic resonance imaging
N	Chemical symbol for nitrogen
Na	Chemical symbol for sodium
NAP	National Association of Phlebotomists
NPSA	National Patient Safety Agency
NRLS	National Reporting and Learning System.
O_2	Chemical symbol for oxygen
Pap	Papanicolaou stain for cervical cell screening

PCO_2	Partial pressure of carbon dioxide
PEP	Post Exposure Prophylaxis
pH	Negative log of hydrogen ion concentration. Below 7 = acid, above 7 = alkali
PICC	Peripherally Inserted Central Catheter
PKU	Phenylketonuria
Plt	Platelets
PO_2	Partial pressure of oxygen
POCT	Point of Care Testing
PPE	Personal Protective Equipment
PRN	As and when required
PSA	Prostate specific antigen
PSA	Professional Standards Authority
PT	Prothrombin time
PTH	Parathyroid hormone
RBC	Red Blood Cell
RFID	Radio Frequency Identification
Rh	Rhesus
SG	Specific gravity
SGOT	Serum Glutamate Oxaloacetate Transaminase
SST	Serum separator tube
STD	Sexually transmitted disease
T_3	Tri-iodothyronine
T_4	Thyroxine
TB	Tuberculosis
TFTs	Thyroid function tests
TP	Total protein
TPN	Total parenteral nutrition
TPR	Temperature, Pulse & Respiration
TSH	Thyroid stimulating hormone
U&E	Urea and Electrolytes
UKAS	United Kingdom Accreditation Service
UTI	Urinary tract infection
UV	Ultraviolet
vCJD	Variant Creutzfeldt-Jakob Disease
VDRL	Venereal Disease Research Laboratory
VLDL	Very low density lipoprotein
VTE	Venous Thrombo-embolism
WBC	White blood cells

Useful Contact Details

Phlebotomy Sampling Systems

BD - Becton-Dickinson (Vacutainer ™)
www.bd.com/uk/

Greiner Bio-One (Vacuette ™)
www.greinerbioone.com/en/england/start/

Kima (Vacutest ™)
info@vacutestkima.it
www.kima.it/

Sarstedt (S – Monovette ™)
Info@sarstedt.com
www.sarstedt.com

National Association of Phlebotomists

The National Association of Phlebotomists was formed in 1995 with the aim of promoting standards in phlebotomy practice to improve patient care, reduce sample errors and raise the profile of phlebotomists with recognition for this valuable skill.

They can be contacted –

E-Mail: phlebotomy@btinternet.com
Website: www.phlebotomy.org

Cord Blood – Stem Cell Collection

Many phlebotomists are now expanding their role by collecting umbilical cord blood samples for harvesting stem cells. These stem cells may be stored publicly or held privately for families. Stem cells can be used to grow and repair new tissues and organs.

This requires taking blood from the umbilical cord and a further sample from the mother. Special training is required and handling and storage of cells is covered by the Human Tissue Authority, Human Tissue Act 2004 and Human Tissue Act (Scotland) 2006.

Further information is available from –

www.cordbloodaware.org

INDEX

ABOUT THE AUTHOR

Roger Hoke has had a long career in healthcare and teaching – both within the hospital and university environment and has a wealth of experience.

Having graduated with an Honours degree in Applied Biomedical Science he proceeded to obtain a Post-Graduate Certificate in Teaching & Learning in Higher Education. He is also a Registered Operating Department Practitioner and sits on the Executive Committee of the National Association of Phlebotomists and is the Editor and co-author of the National Association of Phlebotomists Manual & Practice Portfolio.

Order of Draw

Stopper	Additive	Indications	Inversions
	Tryptic - Soy Protein broth	Blood Cultures Ideally, 10 mls per bottle Aerobic then Anaerobic	3 - 4
	Sodium Citrate 3.2%	INR, APTR, APTT, All Coagulation screening	3 - 4
	Sodium Citrate 3.2%	ESR (Erythrocyte Sedimentation Rate)	3 - 4
	Silica	Viral serology, antibiotic levels	5
	SST gel	All biochemistry, C-RP	5
	Lithium Heparin	Plasma biochemistry Chromosomes	8 – 10
	Potassium EDTA	FBC, HbA1C, Blood Bank, ESR	8 - 10
	EDTA	Blood Bank, Antibody screen Whole blood tests	8 - 10
	Sodium Fluoride / Potassium Oxalate	Fasting Glucose, Glucose tolerance test	8 - 10